# Mnemonics for medical students

Khalid Khan BSc, MRPharm.S, MBBS, MRCGP, DCH, DRCOG, DFFP, DCM
General Medical Practitioner, GP Tutor and Trainer, Croydon, Surrey, UK

ARNOLD
A member of the Hodder Headline Group
LONDON

First published in Great Britain in 2003 by
Arnold, a member of the Hodder Headline Group,
338 Euston Road, London NW1 3BH

**http://www.arnoldpublishers.com**

Distributed in the United States of America by
Oxford University Press Inc.,
198 Madison Avenue, New York, NY10016
Oxford is a registered trademark of Oxford University Press

*British Library Cataloguing in Publication Data*
A catalogue record for this book is available from the British Library

*Library of Congress Cataloging-in-Publication Data*
A catalog record for this book is available from the Library of Congress

ISBN    0340 81114 5

1 2 3 4 5 6 7 8 9 10

Commissioning Editor: Clare Christian
Development Editor: Heather Smith
Project Editor: Wendy Rooke
Production Controller: Lindsay Smith
Cover Design: Amina Dudhia

Typeset in 10 on 12pt Optima by Phoenix Photosetting, Chatham, Kent
Printed and bound in Malta.

What do you think about this book? Or any other Arnold title? Please send your comments to
feedback.arnold@hodder.co.uk

mnemonic /nmnk, ni-/ a. & *n*. M18. [med.L *mnemonicus* f. Gk *mnemonikos* f. *mnemon, mnemon-* mindful, .] ...*adj*. 1 Intended or designed to aid the memory; of or pertaining to mnemonics. Also, (of a formula, code, etc.) easy to remember or understand... 2 Of or pertaining to memory... A mnemonic device, formula, or code.[1]

Please return this book to:

# CONTENTS

# PREFACE: FREQUENTLY ASKED QUESTIONS (FAQS)

For the insatiably curious . . .

**Q. So what exactly is a mnemonic?**

The name comes from the Greek goddess of memory. A mnemonic is essentially any type of memory aid – see above for a more precise definition.

**Q. How is learning somebody else's mnemonic going to help me?**

Given that they have been used for generations, it is plausible that they will actually help. You will remember your own mnemonics best as they will derive from the way your own mind works and will draw on your own particular strengths. However, you can still benefit from somebody else's knowledge or ideas – in fact, that is why you are at university in the first place!

**Q. Well I know people who never used a mnemonic in the whole of their medical career.**

Then you haven't studied your paediatrics! The APGAR score is actually a mnemonic . . . and your first-aid treatment of sprains might be a bit rusty too (see RICE), not to mention a whole host of syndromes, ROY G. BIV for the colours of the spectrum (or you might have used Richard of York Gave Battle In Vain), then there is Every Good Boy Deserves Football for musical sheets, etc. etc.

## Q. Why make revising medicine funny?

Humour is useful as a learning tool – just because something is serious doesn't mean it has to be miserable. Besides, humour coaxes your mind to produce more 'feel good' neurotransmitters, enhancing the learning experience – you are more likely to be interested in something you enjoy. In fact, humour has been used for centuries by doctors who are often exposed daily to the grimmest realities and horrors of human fragility. Humour is a coping and release mechanism, it keeps your sanity and allows you to give your best to your patients.

When a patient first sees you they have no idea of what you have seen or done just before their meeting with you – and neither should they – and they will still expect you to greet them warmly, hopefully with a smile and ideally with a reassuring twinkle in your eye. If you feel good, so will they. (Just try looking totally miserable the next time you see a new patient and see how well that goes!) Peter Ustinov said that comedy is simply a funny way of being serious.

## Q. So things like interest and humour help more than mnemonics?

Exactly.

## Q: The effort of learning these acronyms in the first place makes mnemonics pointless . . . what on earth is SALFOPSM for instance?

AGREED – not all of this type of mnemonic is easy or useful. I have attempted to limit the number of these to a few commonly used ones.

They become more useful if the first *two* letters are used, or if a rhyming word or phonetically similar letter is used – and you will notice plenty of these in this book.

For example **SALFOPSM** is an example of a mnemonic where you have to use a lot of effort learning what the mnemonic means. Although it is used by many students, I thought it was quite difficult.

[However, for the curious, the **branches of the external carotid artery** are: **SALFOPSM**: **S** (**s**uperior thyroid); **A** (posterior **a**uricular); **L** (**l**ingual); **F** (**f**acial); **O** (**o**ccipital); **P** (**p**osterior auricular); **S** (**s**uperior temporal ); **M** (**m**axillary).]

Incidentally the internal carotid is **OPCAM** – I'll let you work it out yourself (sorry).

**Q. Well, I have read about short-term and long-term memory – might memory aids have something to do with this?**

Yes, generally most information enters your 'short-term' memory first and, by an unknown physiological process, is stored permanently as your 'long-term' memory.

All memory aids and systems work by linking your new info. to an already existing piece of memory that you already know. This process of association 'piggy backs' the new knowledge on to the long-term memory.

This means you will assimilate the required knowledge quicker (since your neurons make fewer new physiological changes). Otherwise your brain would be making those neuronal connections the long-winded, tedious and random way.

**Q. So *association* is the basis of having an efficient memory?**

Essentially, yes.

**Q. . . . and you say that physiological changes actually happen when memories are made?**

Yes, the evidence for this has been accumulating for quite some time.

A recent example is that of the brains of London taxi drivers. In March 2000 researchers at University College London scanned the brains of 16 cabbies and found the hippocampus area (important anatomically in memory) had enlarged after 'knowledge' training.

**Q. What about dual-hemisphere brain learning techniques?**

Well, the best way to learn is to utilize both hemispheres of the brain. This bilateral learning is coaxed and encouraged by the use of memory aids. It is inherent in the very nature of mnemonics.

A good mnemonic will make use of the analytical, critical as well as the visual and creative areas of your brain – whether you like it or not.

You will notice already that the *more modalities* you use (e.g. smell, touch, sight, etc.) the easier it is to remember things. The more extreme the sensory input, the more likely you are to remember it. Thus the more vivid the picture, the stronger the smell, the more energetic the associated emotions, the stronger the connotations – the more powerful the memory will be. The memory will more likely to be 'written' directly on to your long-term physiological memory if it is remembered in this way.

**Q. I find that the mnemonics disappear after a while but I don't need them anymore as I just *know* . . .**

Exactly! The facts are now part of your long-term memory – you need mnemonic it no more, know more!

**Q. But all the mnemonics I have heard are rude.**

It doesn't have to be rude or offensive to be useful – although sometimes this helps the associative process. Too many similar phrases will defeat the object of the exercise, so I have not used many of them. Although very popular, they have their limitation as learning tools. Now students are complaining that they are not offensive enough!

**Q. Do you not offend half the students while making the other half giggle?**

Actually the rudest, most offensive and explicit mnemonics were supplied almost entirely by the female medical students. Most were unpublishable, so I haven't, alas, included them here (also because I didn't feel they were particularly good as memory aids, and it also got quite confusing as to who was doing what and how and to whom, etc.).

**Q. I can't find this book in the medical school bookshop.**

Good grief! And this THE most important text there is . . . Quick – give them the publishers details!

**Q. *Hey, can I send you a mnemonic for the next edition – what will I get out of it?***

*Well you will certainly get full credit for your idea or thought, and also a free copy of the next edition.*

**Q. What about any mistakes?**

Said Aeschylus 'the wisest of the wise may err'. So apologies in advance.

These mnemonics do not replace your regular course notes nor do they replace existing or past guidelines or accepted clinical practices. They are for help with revision only, and do not replace clinical judgement or methodology, nor are they a substitute for any part of your training.

Please do send me comments, or point out any of the 'deliberate' mistakes.

**Q. Should I be making notes in the margin, etc.?**

Yes – it will help you to learn.

Jotting and doodling involve more areas of your brain, reinforce the memory and crystallize thoughts in your mind. The process of using your hands as well as both brain hemispheres contributes to whole-brain learning – this will make you a better learner.

**Q. Why do you have so many quotes? Is it to make things interesting?**

Said Confucius: 'Study the past if you would divine the future.'

(Of course another interpretation is that you should look at past papers or ask the students in the year above how they passed last year . . .)

**Q. So as I read and learn, this book, funny yet serious, will be showing me techniques of *association* and how to use *humour* to evoke *interest* and stimulate my neurological memory to its full potential, while giving me the tools to make my own mnemonics and study techniques, and so maximize the efficiency of my revision time?**

Exactly! Well said!

**Q. And there are no rules in mnemonics except to do what works?**

Precisely!

*KK 2003*

# WHY *THIS* BOOK IS SO GOOD

Congratulations! You are a student of one of the most exciting undergraduate courses in the world. Time and knowledge are precious; you are challenged in countless directions with constant syllabus changes . . . and are still expected to have assimilated a colossal amount of raw knowledge.

You need to manage your time and energies efficiently. Herein lies some assistance.

This compilation of medical mnemonics has the emphasis on user-friendliness. Those that are quickest to assimilate are given priority for inclusion, with many popular old favourites. There is guidance on how to study efficiently and create your own memory aids.

You will remember many of them forever – with minimal effort. This book will be there for you all the way from freshers to graduation and beyond . . .

Einstein said that if there is an easier way . . . find it!

There are some easier ways in this magical volume.

Go find 'em!

# ACKNOWLEDGEMENTS

This publication would not have been possible without the help, cooperation and encouragement of hundreds of students from various medical schools. Alas, many innovators of mnemonics over centuries remain anonymous. However, I wish, in particular, to give my thanks to those mentioned below.

| | |
|---|---|
| Aidan Mowbray | Mahmooda Qureshi |
| Amer Shoaib | Mat Jones |
| Aamir Zafar | Megan Morris |
| Andrew Eldridge | Milan Radia |
| Atique Imam | Mike Grocott |
| Azhar Ala | Mr Brown's Rabbit |
| Barry Whitlow | Nazneen Ala |
| Caroline Hallett | Neil Bhatia |
| Chris Menzies | Paul Kennedy |
| Debbie Rogers | Paul McCoubrie |
| Dia Karanough | Paul Roome |
| Dush Mital | Quinn Scobies |
| Hammad Malik | Raj Bhargava |
| Harvey Chant | Raza Toosey |
| Helen Marsden | Dr Robert Clark ('the Barnet course') |

| | |
|---|---|
| John Morlese | 'Rats' |
| Kate Ward | Rob Ward |
| Khalid Hassan | Shahid Khan |
| 'Kuz' | Stuart McCorkel |

Leigh Urwin

The General Management Committee of the St George's Hospital Medical School Club

With extra special thanks to Aftab Ala.

Every effort has been made to trace original sources and copyright holders, but in a compilation such as this it has not always been possible. Any persons who claim copyright should contact the author so that an acknowledgement may be included in future editions.

# Chapter One

# ANATOMY

*Our adventure begins with anatomy – where most students
first come across mnemonics in medicine.*

# THE UPPER LIMB

## The rotator cuff

### SItS

To remember the rotator cuff, think of the word 'SItS'. Looking at the
diagram below you can see how this describes the attachments of the
rotator cuff muscles to the humerus.

Posterior attachments to the humerus:

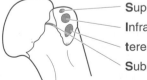

Posterior attachments to the humerus

**S**upraspinatus

**I**nfraspinatus

**t**eres minor (hence little '**t**')

**S**ubscapularis

# The latissimus dorsi

Lady Doris Between Two Majors

An old, anonymous and easy way of remembering that the latissimus dorsi muscle is attached on the humerus; on the floor of the bicipital groove with the tendon between the attachments of pectoralis major and teres major.

# The cubital fossa and Mr Brown's Rabbit

Some students imagine Madeline Brown's Big Red Pustule in order to remember features of the cubital fossa. From **medial to lateral**, embedded in fat, you will find the median nerve, brachial artery, biceps tendon, radial and posterior interosseous nerves:

| | |
|---|---|
| **Madeline** | **median nerve** |
| **Brown's** | **brachial artery** |
| **Big** | **biceps tendon** |
| **Red** | **radial nerve** |
| **Pustule** | **posterior interosseous nerve** |

*Alternatives*

**Mr Brown Bites Rabbits Posteriorly**

**or Madeline Brown's Big Radiology Posting**

**or Madeline Brown's Big Red Pussy**

Disclaimer: The above character is purely fictitious and not based on anybody who ever existed. Mr Brown's rabbit has given the author verbal permission.

# Interossei muscles of the hand

There are four palmar and four dorsal interossei. They all have ulnar nerve innervation.

Thinking of **PAD** and **DAB** will help you remember that:[1]

**Palmar interossei ADduct . . . PAD**

**Dorsal interossei ABduct . . . DAB**

# The carpal bones, Sue and Terry's pens

The eight small bones in the wrist are arranged in two rows of four. Imagine from **lateral to medial**, the proximal row of the wrist (Latin = *carpus*). You see:

scaphoid,

lunate,

triquetral, and

pisiform.

Then visualize the distal row – going the other way – **medial to lateral**:

hamate,

capitate,

trapezoid,

trapezium.

An old favourite for remembering these is one of various versions of:

**Sue Likes Terry's Pens,**

**– Her Cap's Too Tight**

Variations include changing the names, or using alternatives to words such as 'pen' and 'cap', some of which have been too rude to print

[1]*Moore K. 1985:* Clinically orientated anatomy, *2nd edn. Williams & Wilkins.*

here! (Incidentally now is a good time to remind you that the scaphoid, in the snuffbox, is the most commonly shattered bone in the wrist and sometimes not seen on X-ray for some two weeks or so . . . .)

## Alternative

Still too difficult? Try this elegantly fun version in which both rows of carpal bones go from **lateral to medial**:

**Some Lovers Try Positions**
**That They Cannot Handle**

i.e. scaphoid, lunate, triquetral, pisiform (proximal row); trapezium, trapezoid, capitate, hamate (distal row).

Locate on your own wrist to see which one you can remember most easily. The action of locating on your own wrist will reinforce the memory associations in your brain.

# THE THORAX

## Nerve supply to the diaphragm

This simple verse will always be there to remind you that the nerve supply to the diaphragm is via the **3rd, 4th and 5th cervical nerve roots**:

**C**
**three, four and**
**five,**
**keep the diaphragm**
**alive . . .**

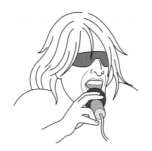

# Costal groove – VAN

The well-known sequence of important structures in the **costal groove** at the inferior border of the rib, going inferiorly, is vein, artery and nerve.

N.B. The rib:

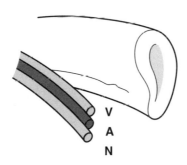

**V**  **vein**

**A**  **artery**

**N**  **nerve**

**in the costal groove.**

# THE ABDOMEN AND PELVIS

## Posterior relations of the kidney

The posterior relations are similar on both sides (the anterior relations are different).

**SWOT BOX**

> There is **one artery** – the subcostal. **Two bones** – 11th and 12th ribs – deep to the diaphragm. There are **three nerves** – the subcostal, iliohypogastric and ilioinguinal – which descend diagonally. Posteriorly, the superior pole of the kidney is related to **four muscles** – the diaphragm, more inferiorly is the quadratus lumborum, medially is the psoas major and laterally the transversus abdominis.

If you remember **'1, 2, 3, 4'** and **'All Boys Need Muscle'** . . .

Now consider the following formula:

| 1 | **artery** | **All** |
|---|---|---|
| 2 | **bones** | **Boys** |
| 3 | **nerves** | **Need** |
| 4 | **muscle** | **Muscle** |

### *Naughty bit*

Cheeky alternative for readers who are a lost cause: **Altered Boys Never Masturbate** or derivatives thereof.

# Renal arteries

To remember the branches of the renal arteries cross your hands in front of you. The thumbs will represent the single posterior segment branch and four fingers = the four main anterior segmental arteries:[2]

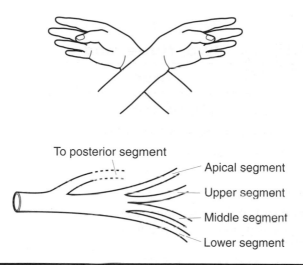

To posterior segment

Apical segment

Upper segment

Middle segment

Lower segment

# The spleen

A useful description of the spleen is that it is **1" × 3" × 5"** in size, it weighs **seven** ounces and lies obliquely between the **9th** and **11th** ribs. To be able to regurgitate all this information, seamlessly, simply remember the sequence:

## 1, 3, 5, 7, 9, 11

[2]From John Blandy 1998: Lecture notes in urology, 5th edn. Oxford: Blackwell Science.

# The anal and urethral sphincters: S2, 3 and 4

Remember that the second, third and fourth sacral nerve roots supply these sphincters. Hence:

**S**

**Two, three, and**

**four,**

**Keep the pee**

**Off the floor**

**!**

## Naughty bit

Some authorities use a suitably shitty word to describe the function of the anal sphincter. Choose what you find most er . . . convenient.

# THE LOWER LIMB

## Adductor muscles of the thigh

There are five adductor muscles of the thigh – **pectineus, gracilis, adductor longus, adductor brevis** and **adductor magnus**. These muscles are all supplied by the **obturator nerve**, except for pectineus (femoral nerve). Part of the adductor magnus is also supplied by the sciatic. They generally originate from the pubis. As well as adducting, they are important in fixating the hip joint and for normal gait.

You will remember this by the olde phrase:

| | |
|---|---|
| **Observe** | **ob**turator |
| **Three Ducks** | **three ad**du**ctors** |
| **Pecking** | **pectineus** |
| **Grass** | **gracilis** |

**SWOT BOX**

- The gracilis (+ its nerves and vessels) may be used surgically to repair damaged muscle.
- A relatively weak muscle, its loss has a minimal effect on leg adduction.
- Incidentally, adductor muscle tears or strains are common in fast bowlers (cricket), whereas ossification of the adductor longus can occur in horse riders.

# Posterior compartment of the thigh

Keith Moore in *Clinically orientated anatomy* mentions how, in ancient times, these muscles (the hamstrings) were slashed to bring down enemy horses and to prevent prisoners running away. Ugh! On a lighter note, here comes Swotty Samantha.[3] It has been suggested that:

| | |
|---|---|
| **Big Fat** | **biceps femoris** |
| **Swotty** | **semitendinous** |
| **Samantha** | **semimembranous** |
| **Ate My** | **adductor magnus** |
| **Hamster's Pens** | **hamstring portion** |

# The lesser sciatic foramen

## No Internals Tonight Padre

This will remind you that the **nerve to obturator internus**, its **tendon** and **pudendal nerve/vessels** pass through here.

[3]*Contributed. Please note that all characters in this booklet are entirely fictional and do not in any way relate to any real persons alive or dead. The only exceptions are those people whose sayings or quotes I have given acknowledgement or credit to. This means that Swotty Samantha is not a real person but a purely fictitious character.*

## Say Grace Before Tea

This elegant memory aid has long been used to remind us that **sartorius** and **gracilis** are attached to the medial surface of the tibia just **before** (i.e. anteriorly to) **semitendinosus** (Anon.).

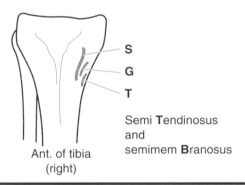

S
G
T

Semi **T**endinosus
and
semimem **B**ranosus

Ant. of tibia
(right)

# Supine or prone?

Any difficulty with these tricky terms is easily resolve with:

## Supine – like a bowl of **soup**

## Prone – like doing **pr**ess-ups.

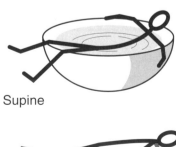

Supine

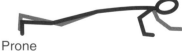

Prone

# Golly, is it a male or a female pelvis?

Look at the greater sciatica notch:

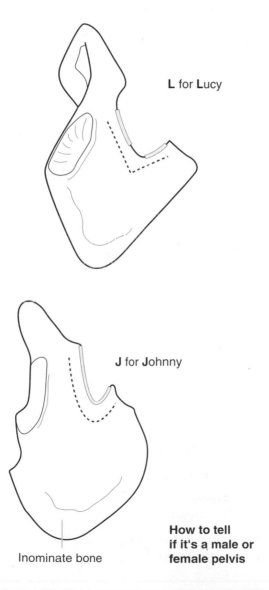

**L** for **L**ucy

**J** for **J**ohnny

Inominate bone

**How to tell
if it's a male or
female pelvis**

# Ankle joint

## Tom, DIck And Harry

Inferior to the medial malleolus lie the tendons of the **t**ibialis posterior, flexor **d**igitorum longus, posterior tibial **a**rtery, posterior tibial **n**erve and flexor **h**allucis longus:[4]

**Right ankle (post.)**

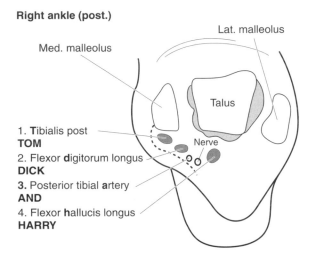

Tom **DI**ck **A**nd **H**arry (Anon.) is said to be a useful mnemonic for remembering positions of tendons around the ANKLE JOINT (very useful in surface anatomy).

## SWOT BOX

- The ankle is the most frequently injured major joint in the body. Nerves: tibial and deep peroneal. The **lateral ligament**, which is the most frequently damaged one, attaches the lateral malleolus to the talus calcaneus.

- Arterial supply to the joint is via the **tibial** arteries (peroneal, anterior and posterior).

[4]See Snell, R.S. 2000: Clinical anatomy for medical students. Little, Brown Medical Division.

It is also worth quoting the second-letter rule for inversion/eversion of the ankle joint (after Robert O'Connor, University College, Dublin):

**Everting muscles are perineus longus/ brevis/terius**

**Inverting muscles are tibialis anterior and posterior.**

# The femoral triangle: NAVY and PIMP

The femoral triangle can be found as a depression inferior to the inguinal ligament (the base of the triangle). Medially is the adductor longus and laterally is the sartorius (more obvious if the thigh is flexed, abducted and laterally rotated).

When you need to take blood via a femoral 'stab' or to perform left cardiac angiographies it is handy to think of NAVY (of course, you do need to know where your Y-fronts are for this to work . . .)

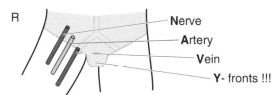

**N  nerve**

**A  artery**

**V  vein**

**Y  Y-fronts**

Meanwhile, going **medial to lateral**, the floor of the triangle consists of the pectineus (P), iliacus (I) and psoas major (MP), giving you

**PIMP.**

**SWOT BOX**

- **Femoral hernias** arise just inferolateral to the pubic tubercle, below the inguinal ligament, medial to the femoral vein.

- Femoral hernias also more common in women, due to the wider pelvis.

# THE HEAD AND NECK

## Layers of the SCALP

This must be a very popular mnemonic judging by the number of texts it is quoted in – and justifiably so.

| | |
|---|---|
| **S** | **skin** |
| **C** | **connective tissue** |
| **A** | **aponeurosis** |
| **L** | **loose connective tissue** |
| **P** | **periosteum** |

## Foramen magnum . . . limp sympathetic men wear corduroy accessories

The important structures passing through are:

- meningeal **lymp**hatics,
- **sympathetic** plexus (on the vertebral arteries),
- **men**inges,
- **ver**tebral arteries (+ spinal branches),

- the spinal **cord**,

- **accessory** nerves . . .

## Limp, Sympathetic Men Vear Corduroy Accessories

– helpful in a clinch. (No apologies if it isn't!)

# Foramina of Luschka and Magendie

The **roof of the fourth ventricle** has **three foramina** – the medial foramen of Magendie and the two foramina of Luschka. The cerebrospinal fluid leaves via these openings into the subarachnoid space.

## Magendie is medial

## Luschka is lateral[5]

# Four middle cranial holes: a superior orbital fissure . . .

The structures passing through are the nerves:

- lacrimal,

- frontal,

- trochlear,

- superior division of III,

- oculomotor (n. to superior oblique),

- nasociliary nerve,

- inferior division of III, and

- abducens (VI).

[5]Liebman M. Neuroanatomy made easy and understandable, 4th edn. University Park Press.

| Lazy | lacrimal |
| French | frontal |
| Tarts | trochlear |
| Sprawl | sup. Div. III (n. to sup. oblique) |
| Naked | nasociliary |
| In | inf div of III |
| Anticipation | abducens |

## SWOT BOX

The superior orbital fissure lies between the lateral wall and the roof of the orbit. It allows structures to communicate with the middle cranial fossa; a penetrating injury to the eye can therefore enter the middle cranial fossa and the frontal lobe.

The superior orbital fissure meets the inferior orbital fissure at the apex of the orbit. The other three main middle cranial fossa openings are the foramen rotundum, ovale and spinosum (**ROS**). The first two are in the greater wing of the sphenoid, the latter near the spine of the sphenoid (hence its name, 'spinosum').

# ... and three other foramina

## Max Returns Mandy's Ovum
## – (May Marry a Spinster)

Thinking about Max Returning Mandy's Ovum is a neat way to remind yourself that the **max**illary nerve exits the skull via the foramen rotundum, and the **mand**ibular nerve via the foramen **ov**ale.

You also add 'May Marry a Spinster' to remind you that the important **m**iddle **m**eningeal **ar**tery passes through the foramen **spin**osum.

# Four parasympathetic ganglia

How to remember that the four parasympathetic ganglia are **c**iliary, **o**tic, **p**terygopalatine and **s**ub-mandibular?

Well you can try:

## COPS

If this is far too boring, and you are not the politically correct type, then perhaps the rather unflattering phrase, Silly Old People Stay Mouldy, will help.

| | |
|---|---|
| **Silly** | **ciliary** |
| **Old** | **otic** |
| **People** | **pterygopalatine** |
| **Stay Mouldy** | **sub-mandibular** |

## SWOT BOX

- The ciliary ganglion is in the posterior orbit – the oculomotor nerve (III) goes here. Post-ganglionic fibres supply ciliary muscles and pupils.
- The hypoglossal (IX) nerve supplies the otic ganglion and connects to the parotid gland, causing salivation.
- The pterygopalatine (or sphenopalatine) ganglion lies in its own fossa; nerve fibres come from the facial nerve (VII) and thence supply the lacrimal, nasal and palatine glands.
- The submandibular ganglion has fibres from the facial nerve (VII). It supplies the sublingual and (you guessed it) the submandibular gland.

# The circle of Willis

Often students find it helpful to think in terms of a spider visualization:[6]

## Have you met Willis the spider?

He has a face

Eight legs

And a Willis...!

See next page for all else to be revealed . . .

[6]*From Goldberg*, Clinical neuroanatomy made ridiculously simple. *MedMaster, 2003.*

### 'Willis the spider'

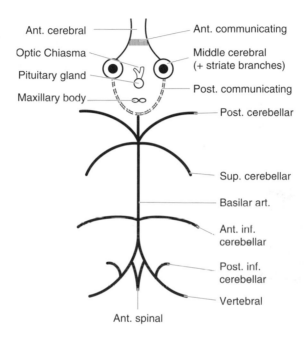

Remember the exam favourite . . . pontine branches.

# External carotid artery

## SALFOPSM

I didn't feel that this was an especially good mnemonic; however, as it is undoubtedly used by some students, I've mentioned it in the Preface (FAQs).

# Carotid sheath: NAVY or AJAX

This is a portion of tubular cervical fascia enclosing the vagus nerve, carotid artery and internal jugular vein.

AJAX is a quick way to remember what is in it:

**A**     **artery no. 1 – common carotid**

**J**     **jugular vein**

**A**     **artery no. 2 – the internal carotids**

**X**     **Xth cranial nerve, the vagus**

### Alternative

NAVY works as a useful formula if used like this:

**N**     **nerve: the vagus**

**A**     **arteries: common and internal carotids**

**V**     **vein: the internal jugular**

**Y**     **the common carotid has two terminal branches – this resembles the letter Y**

**SWOT BOX**

> Incidentally, the sheath extends from the base of the skull to the thorax. If these large blood vessels are moved during surgery, the vagus will be moved with them.

# The cranial nerves

| Is it **S**ensory, **M**otor or **B**oth? | | Learn the names:[7] |
|---|---|---|
| **I.** | **S**ome | **I O**lfactory | **O**n |
| **II.** | **S**ay | **II O**ptic | **O**ld |
| **III.** | **M**arry | **III O**culomotor | **O**lympus |
| **IV.** | **M**oney | **IV T**rochlear | **T**owering |
| **V.** | **B**ut | **V T**rigeminal | **T**op |
| **VI.** | **M**y | **VI A**bducens | **A** |
| **VII.** | **B**ride | **VII F**acial | **F**inn |
| **VIII.** | **S**ays | **VIII V**estibulocochlear | **W**ith a |
| **IX.** | **B**ig | **IX G**lossopharyngeal | **G**erman |
| **X.** | **B**alls | **X V**agus | **V**iewed |
| **XI.** | **M**atter | **XI A**ccessory | **A** |
| **XII.** | **M**ore | **XII H**ypoglossal | **H**ouse |

## Naughty bit

However, most students seem to have gone for:

### Oh Oh Oh To Touch and Feel Virgin Girls' Vaginas and Hymens.

[7]Modified from *Norman Browse 1997*: An introduction to signs and symptoms of surgical disease, *3rd edn. London: Arnold.*

The author feels that the most powerful way to learn this list is via a Peg mnemonic (see Chapter 10, p. 129).

# CRANIAL NERVES AND THE EYE

## Cranial nerves

The **superior oblique** muscle is innervated by the **4th cranial nerve**. Think:

### SO4.

The **lateral recti** are supplied by the **6th nerve** (abducens, which abduct the eye). Think:

### LR 6.

**All** other extra-ocular eye muscles are innervated by the **3rd nerve** (oculomotor). So if you remember the formula:

### LR 6 (SO4) 3

You now know the entire cranial innervations of the extra-ocular eye muscles – Oh you little genius![8]

### RUDE RIDDLE

Why is an Argyll Robertson pupil like a prostitute?

Answer: because it accommodates but doesn't react!

[8]Derived from Smith A. 1972: Irving's anatomy mnemonics. Edinburgh: Churchill Livingstone.

# Branches of the facial (VII) nerve

## Two Zebras Buggered My Cat

| | |
|---|---|
| **Two** | **t**emporal |
| **Z**ebras | **z**ygomatic |
| **B**uggered | **b**uccal |
| **M**y | **m**andibular |
| **C**at | **c**ervical |

---

### RUDE RIDDLE

What do the chorda tympani (facial n. branch) and the clitoris have in common?

(For the answer turn to the next page!)

(The action reinforces the information you are about to learn.)

---

# Vestibulocochlear (VIII)

Thinking of **COWS** helps to remind one of a test for the vestibular division of the VIIth nerve, involving pouring cold or warm water into the external auditory meatus (ear hole!).

The temperature change affects movement of endolymph in the semicircular ducts. This stimulates the cristae hair cells (movement sensors). The vestibular nerve is now stimulated and, via the oculogyric nuclei in the brainstem, will cause **nystagmus**.

**Cold** water causes nystagmus in the direction of the **opposite** eye, **warm** water in the direction of the **same** eye.

**C    cold**

**O    opposite**

**W    warm**

**S    same**

## SWOT BOX

Remember, the direction on nystagmus is that of the 'quick' flick. In nystagmus the eye wanders off, out of control. The brain attempts to correct by flicking the eye back into position so it can fixate on the object being looked at.

## RUDE RIDDLE

Answer to chorda tympani rude riddle: they both supply taste to the anterior two-thirds of the tongue . . . awful! (Anon., not surprisingly!)

# Course of the oculomotor nerve (III)

I know it is a bit of a mouthful, but no mnemonics book would be complete without at least one verse/song. Below is from *Irving's Anatomy Mnemonics* by Alastair Smith (1972) (probably written pre-1939):

**Through peduncular cistern first I run,**

**Then pierce dura – just for fun;**

**Here posterior clinoid is to medium**

**Between two borders of tentorium**

**Next laterally to the sinus I go,**

**Crossed by trochlear from below;**

**Into two branches then I split**

**And this round nasociliary fit.**

**Thro' orbital fissure next I pass**

**Between heads of lateral rectus**

**Entering orbit that I may**

**Supply levator palpebrae,**

**Inferior oblique and recti three,**

**With twig to the ganglion come from me.**[9,10]

[9]*Verse or songs are a common memory aid. The tradition of using songs to impart knowledge seems to have atrophied somewhat in Europe. In Chinese medical schools, songs are a common way of learning material, and have been for centuries.*
[10]*Reprinted from* Irving's Anatomy Mnemonics, *Alastair Smith, © 1972, with permission from Elsevier.*

Make notes – it will help you to learn

# Chapter Two

# NEUROLOGY AND NEUROSCIENCE

*As well as helping you with the dermatomes, you will be able to cruise through the following:*

## Pre-quiz

- Which fibres carry crude touch?
- Which modalities are carried in dorsal columns?
- Which nerve roots are affected if there is an absent biceps jerk?
- What are the main causes of peripheral neuropathy?
- What are the main causes of mononeuritis multiplex?
- What are the signs of a cerebellar lesion?
- What are the signs of a lesion on the angular gyrus of the dominant hemisphere?
- Which dermatomes do you know?

*More brain, O Lord, more brain!*

*George Meredith*

# Bits of the brain[1]

| | |
|---|---|
| **T**oddlers' | **t**elencephalon |
| **M**essy | **m**esencephalon |
| **D**iapers | **d**iencephalon |
| **T**urn | **m**etencephalon |
| **Y**ellow | **m**yencephalon |

# Ventral and dorsal spinal columns

To remember that the grey ventral columns are motor, simply be aware that:

## the motor is in the front of most cars

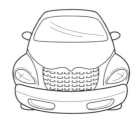

**Sensory**

**Modalities are**

**Dorsal**

[1]Debbie Rogers.

Well if you find the above too simple, then for further challenges look at Julie's Visible Panty Line:

| | |
|---|---|
| **Julie's** | **joint position** |
| **Visible** | **vibration** |
| **Panty** | **pressure** |
| **Line** | **light touch** |

# C-fibres carry crude touch

## 'C' is for 'Crude'

---

**SWOT BOX**

C-fibres are involved with pain that typically arises slowly, is poorly localized, often a burning and unpleasant or disagreeable sensation.

---

# A-fibres

## (Pain) arises abruptly, is blocked by asphyxia – the As.

**SWOT BOX**

A-fibres are involved with pain that arises abruptly, is well localized, often sharp or prickling.

(Come to think of it, they have a lot in common with getting 'A' grades too.)

# Reflexes

A popular and simple aide-memoir:[2]

| Ankle  | S1, 2 |
|--------|-------|
| Knee   | L3, 4 |
| Biceps | C5, 6 |
| Triceps| C7, 8 |

**SWOT BOX**

All the muscles on the dorsal aspect of the upper limb are innervated by C7. In other words, the triceps, wrist and finger extensors.

# Dermatomes made easier

Imagine (to switch on the right side of your brain!) a four-legged mammal rather than a biped – this makes understanding the dermatomes much easier.

[2]After Rubenstein and Wayne Lecture notes in clinical medicine, 4th edn. Oxford: Blackwell Scientific.

Start at **C1** and work your way down . . . **C1 to C4** are the head/neck shoulders then **C5 to T1** 'disappear' as they wander off to innervate the upper limb.

You know that **T4 supplies the nipples** and **T10 the umbilicus** (see below if you don't ).

**T12 is the lowest abdominal dermatome** and after this **L1 to S1** go to the lower limb. This leaves **S2 to S5** for the bottom end.

If you study the following diagram and transpose it to a biped, you will see the way the dermatomes flow. Go with that flow!

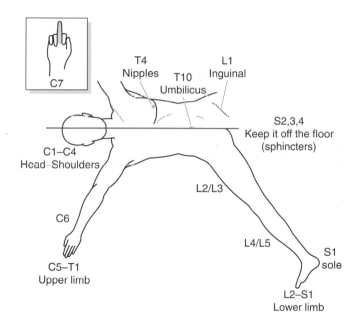

## RUDE RIDDLE

Which dermatome innervates the nipples?

See below.

# *T10 Dermatome: the umbilicus*

Did you know that the umbilicus is already **labelled** with its respective dermatome?

Not convinced? Do I have to draw you a diagram?

OK here it is . . . but for the **rest of your life you will remember that T10 innervates the umbilicus . . .**

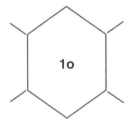

## RUDE RIDDLE

Answer to rude riddle: T4 ('T for (4) tits').

Another useful way of looking at dermatomes:[3]

## You stand on S1

## Lie on S2

## Sit on S3

## Wipe S4

## Poke S5 (PR)

[3]*Contributed by Dr Laura Colvin.*

## More dermatomes . . .

**One cervical, two cervical, three cervical, four**

**Down the upper limb to find any more,**

**Hold out your arms like a crucifix,**

**Stick up your thumbs – you have C6;**

**Now wiggle C7 – the middle finger – to heaven;**

**And easy to extrapolate**

**Ring and little fingers are C8!**

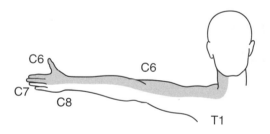

The dermatome to the axilla is T1 (remember the overlap of all dermatomes).

T1 is actually spelt in **armp 1T**:

### armp 1T

1L is spelt in **1nguinaL** – picture this and it will remind you of the dermatome of the inguinal area.

### 1nguina L

Also:

**L3 goes to medial knee
(rhymes)
S1 – one Small toe**

The first sacral nerve supplies the little toes – get it?

You have now learned, with minimal effort, most of the major dermatomes.

Once you know a few key dermatomes you can extrapolate the rest.

Remember **all dermatomes overlap** with the ones above and below, which makes revision even easier!

Review them in the 'Dermatome Song' below – remember that reviewing is the key to success.

## *Dermatome song*

**One cervical, two cervical, three cervical, four**

**Down the upper limb to find any more,**

**Hold out your arms like a crucifix,**

**Stick up your thumbs – you have C6;**

**Now wiggle C7 – the middle finger to heaven;**

**And easy to extrapolate**

**Ring and little fingers are C8!**


**T1 spelt in 'Armp 1T' is,**

**As for nipples, well T (4) for 'tits'**

**One dermatome ready labelled for us**
**T10 in the umbilicus!**

**1L, spelt in '1nguinaL',**
**With L3 to medial knee**
**L4 goes across your kneecap**
**But won't stop there, the busy chap!**
**It goes to make your bunion tingle**
**And with L5 the big toe jingle!**

**S1 (upon which you stand) ends in *one***
***Small* toe**
**S2 on which you lie**
**S3 upon which you sit**
**S4 is what you wipe**
**S5 – put yer finger innit!**

OK so it is a little dire in places – but at least you know more dermatomes than you did ten minutes ago!

# Causes of peripheral neuropathy[4]

**A**    alcohol

**B**    $B_{12}$

**C**    CRF and Ca

**D**    diabetes and drugs

**E**    every vasculitis

# Mononeuritis multiplex

**SCALD** will remind you of causes . . .

**S**    sarcoid

**C**    Ca

**A**    arteritis

**L**    leprosy

**D**    diabetes

# Gerstmann's syndrome

### A-ALF

This is a combination of :

     **a**graphia,

     **a**calculia,

     **l**eft/right disorientation,

     **f**inger agnosia.

[4]After Dr R. Clarke Medicine for Finals: reproduced with permission from the excellent revision course conducted by Dr Clarke of Barnet General Hospital /Chase Farm Hospitals Trust.

**SWOT BOX**

This is due to a lesion in the angular gyrus of the dominant hemisphere.

- **Agraphia** means the inability to write.
- **Acalculia** is similar, but for simple arithmetic calculations.
- **Agnosia** is the loss of recognition of sensory stimuli.

*Josef Gerstmann, Vienna neurologist (1887–1969)*

# Cerebellar signs – DANISH[5]

Popular in exams! It is definitely worth knowing the following mnemonic well.

**D** **dysdiadochokinesia**

**A** **ataxia**

**N** **nystagmus**

**I** **intention tremor, ~ 3 Hz**

**S** **speech (scanning/stoccato)**

**H** **hypotonia**

[5]After Dr R. Clarke *Medicine for Finals: reproduced with permission from the excellent revision course conducted by Dr Clarke of Barnet General Hospital /Chase Farm Hospitals Trust.*

**SWOT BOX**

- Cerebellar signs are **ipsilateral** to a lesion.

- **Dysdiadochokinesia** is impairment in the ability to perform rapidly alternating movements, e.g. sequential supination and pronation.

- **Ataxia** (Greek, *taxis* = order; *a* = negative) is lack of muscular coordination, *and* leads to an abnormal gait. The patient often staggers and walks with a broad-based gait for stability, and tends to fall in the direction of the side of the lesion.

- Cerebellar **nystagmus** is usually horizontal (ask patient to look laterally). Use 'finger–nose' test to show the 'past-pointing' effect of the **intention tremor** (e.g. when asked to touch the nose the patient misses and hits the cheek). Note that tremor is not affected by closing the eyes and occurs during a movement, not at rest (unlike Parkinson's disease).

- **Speech** is often affected (dysarthria), sometimes described as 'slurred and explosive'.

- The muscles are **often hypotonic** but may also be hypertonic. This, of course, aggravates the ataxia.

# Causes of abnormal gait

**All Patients Spending Cash See Proper Doctors**

| **All** | **apraxia/ataxia** |
| **Patients** | **parkinsonism** |

| Spending | spasticity |
| Cash | cerebellar ataxia |
| See | sensory deficit |
| Proper | proximal myopathy |
| Doctors | distal myopathy |

### SWOT BOX

Apraxia is the inability to perform learned voluntary movements in the absence of paralysis. If this involves loss of writing ability, it is called agraphia.

# Epileptic seizure

**The aura, the cry**

**The fall, the fit**

**The tonus, the clonus,**

**The piss and the shit.**

**Describes an epileptic fit.**

Note: this obviously gives useful features of a tonic (spasm)/clonic (jerking) seizure. Where this is useful is that it helps differentiating whether the fit was epileptiform or not.

You do, of course, need to be aware of the wide variety of clinical patterns of epilepsy, which includes altered motor and sensory phenomena, altered consciousness and sometimes odd behaviour.

Make notes – it will help you to learn

# Chapter Three

# BIOCHEMISTRY

*Some tips and suggestions to help with biochemistry revision:*

## Pre-quiz

- How many rings are there in the adenine nucleotide?
- Which are the pyrimidine nucleotide bases?
- How many hydrogen bonds are there between guanine and cytosine?
- What are the four fates of pyruvate?
- Draw the Lineweaver–Burke plot showing competitive inhibition.
- Draw an α-helix.
- Name the essential amino acids – how many of them are there?

# GALA – The four fates of pyruvate

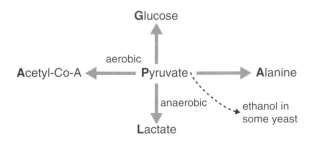

# Lineweaver–Burke plot of enzyme inhibition

Compare the graph of competitive inhibition with this visual memory aid of two crossed swords:

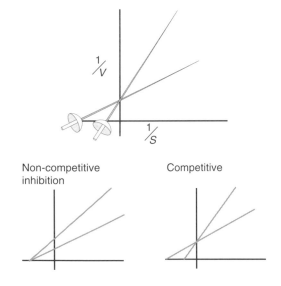

# The 12 essential amino acids

**Meeting Three Argentine Sisters**

**Like Lucy, Tracy and Val;**

**His Phone Is so Tired**

| | |
|---|---|
| **M**eeting | **m**ethionine |
| **T**hree | **t**hreonine |
| **A**rgentine | **a**rginine |
| **S**isters | **c**ysteine |
| **L**ike | **l**ysine |
| **L**ucy | **l**eucine |
| **T**racy and | **t**yrosine |
| **V**al | **v**aline |
| **H**is | **h**istidine |
| **P**hone (or 'Pen') | **p**henylalanine |
| **I**s so | **i**soleucine |
| **T**ired | **t**yrosine |

### *Alternative*

Well I suppose

**Any Help In Learning These Tiny Little Molecules Could Prove Truly Valuable**

may be used instead, if you wish . . . yawn.

# Lipids

VLDLs (very-low-density lipoproteins) carry triglycerides from hepatic to peripheral and other cells, where they are stored and later used for metabolism.

HDLs (high-density lipoproteins) carry cholesterol away from the peripheral cells to the liver for excretion.

Think:

**H for Heroes**

**and**

**V for Villains**

# Oxidation and reduction

There is of course the old school favourite:

**OILRIG**

**Oxidation is loss and reduction is gain (of electrons).**

# Purines and pyrimidines

**All Girls Are Pure and Wear Bras**

Nucleic acids are made up of a base, a five-carbon sugar and a phosphate group. The bases are either the purines (two-ringed) adenine and guanine, whereas the pyrimidines are the single-ringed thymine and cytosine (or uracil in RNA). Within the nucleic acid chain, a pyrimidine always links with a purine and vice versa. So a DNA double helix is *always* three rings wide.

## *Adenine and guanine are purines*

**All adenine and**

**Girls**          **guanine**

**are Pure**       **are purines**

## *Purines are two-ringed structures*

. . . and so are bras!

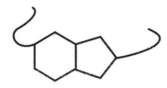

## *This leaves the single ringed pyrimidines, thymine and cytosine*

Perhaps you can think of Pies (single ring shape); or Tyres and Cytes (cells) are single ringed, so perhaps that will help.

Or you can imagine a 'seat' for cytosine.

Get the picture? If not, make your own – *you are more likely to remember your own mental pictures than somebody else's.*

And your memory likes to work in pictures.

**Penser, c'est voir:** *To think is to see.*

*Louis Lambert*

# Base pairing at the GEC

You will remember that a purine only pairs with a pyrimidine (giving a constant three-ring diameter to DNA).

- Adenine only pairs with thymine, think

**AT**

- Guanine links with cytosine (via three hydrogen bonds). This is ridiculously easy to remember if you think of the General Electric Company – GEC . . .

**G≡C**

# Protein structure: how to draw an α-helix

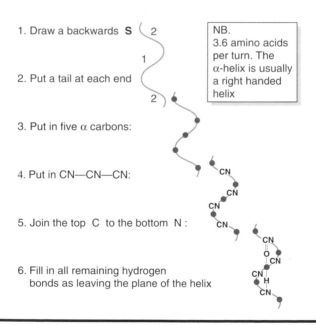

1. Draw a backwards **S**

2. Put a tail at each end

3. Put in five α carbons:

4. Put in CN—CN—CN:

5. Join the top C to the bottom N :

6. Fill in all remaining hydrogen bonds as leaving the plane of the helix

NB.
3.6 amino acids per turn. The α-helix is usually a right handed helix

# The urea cycle

I am assured by several students that this actually helped them with the urea cycle. There is no accounting for taste . . .

| | |
|---|---|
| **O**rdinarily | **o**rnithine |
| **C**areless | **c**arbamoyl PO$_4$ |
| **C**rappers | **c**itrulline |
| **A**re | **a**spartate |
| **A**lso | **a**rginosuccinate |
| **F**rivolous | **f**umarate |
| **A**bout | **a**rginine |
| **U**rination | **u**rea         **Anon.** |

(The biochemical cycles are probably best learnt by use of loci or peg mnemonics – see Chapter 10).

# Fat-soluble vitamins

**ADEK**

Make notes – it will help you to learn

# Chapter Four

# PHYSIOLOGY AND PHARMACOLOGY

## Pre-quiz

- Which are the five main excretory organs?
- Are $\beta_1$ receptors found predominantly in lung or heart?
- How many litres of interstitial fluid in an average adult?
- Is ejaculation parasympathetic or sympathetic?
- How is arterial blood pressure defined?
- What effect does constriction of the iris have on the canal of Schlemm?
- Is the above sympathetic or parasympathetic?
- What are the components of S1?
- Draw a sarcomere (just for fun!).
- Is phenytoin used in the treatment of petit mal?
- Which prostaglandins dilate blood vessels?

# PHYSIOLOGY
## Arterial blood pressure

### BP Copper

Thinking **BP Copper** reminds one that

BP = CO × PR

**BP   arterial blood pressure**
**CO   cardiac output**
**PR   peripheral resistance**

---

*Boredom is a sign of satisfied ignorance, blunted apprehension, crass sympathies, dull understanding, feeble powers of attention and irreclaimable weakness of character.*
                                        *James Bridle (Mr Bolfry)*

*So keep your mind occupied with useful, productive things, which are funny, make you feel good AND get you more marks with less effort – like making up mnemonics – just a suggestion! Look for any patterns in the stuff you need to remember; however weird and illogical, so long as they make some sense to you it will probably work. At the very least you will be more familiar with the material.*
                                        *K Khan*

(And if it is a good one so we can mention you in the next edition!)

# Those six anterior pituitary hormones

The six anterior pituitary hormones are:

> thyroid stimulating hormone (TSH),
>
> growth hormone (GH);
>
> the gonadotrophins, follicle stimulating hormone (FSH) and luteinizing hormone (LH),
>
> prolactin, and
>
> adrenocorticotrophic hormone (ACTH).

| Those Giant Gonads Prolong the Action | |
|---|---|
| Those | TSH |
| Giant | GH |
| Gonads | gonadotrophins (LH/FSH) |
| Prolong | prolactin |
| the Action | ACTH |

# Immunoglobulins – GAMED

There are five classes of immunoglobulins – Ig **G, A, M, E** and **D**. Each has four polypeptide chains – two heavy and two light. The chains are held together by disulphide bonds. Heavy chains are specific to each class of Ig.

IgM is produced first in the immune response. Later IgG appears as the IgM levels fall. IgG forms the secondary response, which is due to activation of long-lived B-cells on repeat exposure to the antigen. The secondary response is quicker and greater than the primary response.

Remember :

**IgM is produced iMMediately**

**IgG response is the Greater**

# Point and Shoot[1]

**PARASYMPATHETIC SYMPATHETIC**
**(→; erection)          (→; ejaculation)**

(Surely you don't need a diagram for this one.)

# Fluid compartment formula[2]

This one needs a little bit of thinking (stay calm – it's not too much). You need to say to yourself: **1,2,3,30,45 – IF.PIT**. It works something like this:

| | |
|---|---|
| **12 litres of interstitial fluid (IF)** | **1 2** |
| **3 litres of plasma (P)** | **3** |
| **30 litres inside cells (I)** | **30** |
| **Total (T)** | **45** |
| **IF.PIT** | |

Well, yes, maybe it is a little painful at first but do have a go, I'm sure you'll like it when you get used to it. No, it isn't one of mine – it was contributed by a medical student. Write it out a few times (NOW) and you will remember it. Writing will reinforce a motor memory and sensory pathway to strengthen the visual stimulus of the above. Now go do it.

# SKILLED with the excretory organs?

A **SKILL** worth knowing . . . skin, kidneys, intestines, liver, lungs, the five main excretory organs.

[1]With acknowledgement to P. McCoubrie and M. Jones 1990, St Georges' Hospital Medical School.
[2]Contributed by A. Iman (1987, SGHMS) FRCS.

# Beta Receptors

There are $\beta_1$ receptors on the heart;

There are $\beta_2$ receptors on the lung.

## You have ONE heart ($\beta$-ONE) and TWO lungs ($\beta$-TWO).

Does it *get* much easier?

# CCCP

**Constriction of**

**Circular muscle opens up the**

**Canal of Schlemm**

**Parasympathetically**

## SWOT BOX

- Friedrich S. Schlemm (1795–1858) was Professor of Anatomy in Berlin.

- The canal is a space at the sclero-corneal junction; it drains the aqueous fluid away from the anterior chamber. Any increased resistance to this flow will cause a rise in intra-ocular pressure (IOP).

- Schlemm was *over 21* when he discovered the canal. By a freak coincidence, an IOP of *over 21 mmHg* is a sign of glaucoma.

*Gotcha...!*

Now for the rest of your medical career you will know that an *IOP > 21* is a sign of glaucoma – whether you ever wanted to or not!

## RAPID EYE REVISION

- Which eye muscles are innervated by the IIIrd cranial nerve?
- Why is the Argyll Robertson pupil like a prostitute?
- Give some other characteristics of syphilis.

You will know all of these from the section on cranial nerves and the eye (p. 22) and also p. 66 (syphilis).

# Heart sounds made easy

## Mighty Ape

The first heart sound (S1) is made up of a mitral component (M1) and a tricuspid (T1) component (in order of valve closure).

S2 is made up of A2 (aortic) followed by the pulmonary valve closure (P2).

This gives:

S1      S2

M1 T1   A2 P2

Beginners will find this sequence easy with

## Mighty Ape
## i.e. M1 T1, A2 P2

See p. 80 for more heart sounds.

# Khalid's guide to the sarcomere

1. Draw two 'Z lines' – the borders of our 'Zarcomere'.

2. Draw an 'M' line in the Middle.

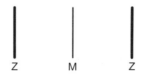

3. Add a dArk 'A' bAnd.

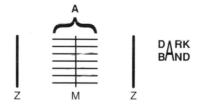

4. What's left must be the lIght 'I' zone.

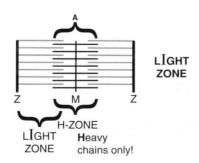

Simple!

# PHARMACOLOGY

## α/β receptors revisited

The phrase:

### β makes 'em bigger

will remind one that β-stimulation generally dilates structures that are lined with smooth muscle, e.g. bronchioles, uterus, blood vessels.

Also, if you imagine the letter α in the shape of a knot:

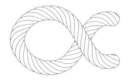

which, when pulled, gets tighter, you may perhaps remember that α-stimulation →; constriction!

---

## RAPID REVISION: βRECEPTORS – ONE HEART AND TWO LUNGS

The heart has predominantly $\beta_1$ sympathetic receptors; the lungs are mainly $\beta_2$.

Remember **ONE heart** (β-ONE) and **TWO lungs** (β-TWO).

# Prostaglandins

Prostaglandins I$_2$, A, E are vasodilators. Think of:

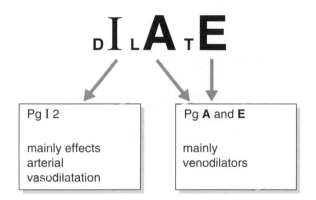

Pg I 2

mainly effects
arterial
vasodilatation

Pg **A** and **E**

mainly
venodilators

# The structure of 6-aminopenicillamic acid

6-APA – the basis of the penicillins!

1. Draw a house:

2. Add a garage and smoke from the chimney:

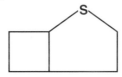

3. Add an outdoor aerial and a garden fence:

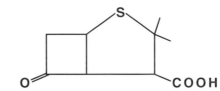

4. Stick on an amide group:

Congratulations!

# Depression – seven 'A's

**A**nhedonia

**A**ppetite loss

**A**nergia

**a**m waking

**A**menorrhoea

**A**sexual ($\downarrow$ libido)

**A**ffective disorder

# Some drugs with zero-order kinetics

**Constantly Aspiring to Phone Ethan**

| **Constantly** | zero-order kinetics |
|---|---|
| **Aspiring** | **aspirin** |
| to **P**hone | **phenytoin** |
| **Ethan** | **ethanol** |

# Petit mal – the paradoxical Ps

Phenytoin, primidone and phenobarbitone are NOT used for petit mal epilepsy. This is the observation of the paradoxical Ps:

**If it starts with a P it ain't used for petit mal!**

**SWOT BOX**

- Petit mal or absence seizures are brief, with a particular ~3 Hz spike-wave pattern; on EEG they are generalized seizures.

- Usually occur between ages 4 and 12 years, characterized by lapses of concentration, some rhythmic movements of eyelids and hands. There is rapid return to full consciousness without retrograde amnesia or confusion.

- Many patients later develop generalized tonic–clonic seizures

- Current treatment involves use of valproate and ethosuximide.

## SWOT TRIVIA BOX

- Phenytoin is a barbiturate. These were named after 'Barbara' (a waitress in Munich) and 'urea'. It is believed by some that Barbara supplied some of the raw materials required.[3]

- The anti-epileptic drug vigabatrin was named after its mode of action (i.e. via GABA-transferase inhibition).

- Another interesting anticonvulsant is clobazam (Rivotril®), which seems to describe the action in knocking patients out (say it quickly). Likewise, the analgesic Dolobid® is named after dolor (pain of inflammation) and the bid dose (twice daily).

- Lasix® (frusemide) was named thus because it 'lasts six hours'.

See, it helps to talk to the drug rep sometimes!

# TB treatment

RIPE and DOT – see Chapter 5.

[3]Sharpless, S.K. 1965: The barbiturates. In The pharmacological basis of therapeutics, 3rd edn. New York: Macmillan, 105–28.

Make notes – it will help you to learn

# Chapter Five

# MICROBIOLOGY AND INFECTIOUS DISEASE

*When you have read this chapter you will be able to tackle the following.*

## Pre-quiz

- List the complications of mumps.
- Is *Neisseria* a Gram-negative or -positive organism?
- Do shigella have flagella, making them motile?
- What is the quadruple therapy of tuberculosis?
- List some non-lactose fermenters.
- List some of the features of syphilis.

## Moping about mumps?

**Meningism**

**Orchitis/Oophoritis**

**Parotitis/Pancreatitis/Paramyxovirus**

**Encephalitis**

## SWOT BOX

- Mumps is an airborne paramyxovirus (also spread by direct contact via body fluids).

- Uncommon in adults, it is often subclinical in children.

- Usually salivary gland inflammation is the principal manifestation, e.g. parotitis (uni- or bilateral).

- Complications include epididymo-orchitis, oophoritis, meningo-encephalitis and pancreatitis.

- Mumps meningitis is usually benign (vomiting, neck rigidity, lethargy, headache, photophobia, convulsions, abdominal pain and fever).

# RNA viruses

## It is no coincidence (?) most RNA viruses start with the letter R . . .

Consider Rhabdovirus (e.g. rabies), Reovirus, Rotavirus, Rhinovirus . . . and a drug with a VIR is often antiviral (think of Retrovir®, Zovirax® and Vectavir®).

# 'Neisseria are negative cocci Sugar'

Microbiologists use cultures containing glucose and maltose in order to differentiate between the negative cocci *N. meningitides* and *N. gonorrhoeae*.

*Neisseria gonorrhoeae* ferments glucose only, whereas *Neisseria meningitides* ferments **glucose and maltose**.

**This is called the sugar fermentation test.**

> ***N. gonorrhoeae* ferments glucose only**
>
> ***N. meningitides* ferments maltose as well.**

# Salmonella and shigella

Both organisms are important in food poisoning. They are both non-lactose fermenters.

Salmonella are flagellate organisms and motile, whereas shigella have no flagella and are therefore non-motile. Can you remember which one is motile? Well you can easily . . . if you think of a salmon!

Yes, a salmon . . . if you can remember that salmon are motile, then you will know that **salmonella are motile** too!

Your space to draw picture of a salmon:

Remember the following non-lactose fermenters:

## SSPP

**salmonella, shigella, *Pseudomonas*, *Proteus*.**

# Syphilis

**There was a young lad from Bombay,**

**Whose chancre just wouldn't fade away,**

**Well apart from his tabes,**

**And sabre-legged babies,**

**Now he thinks he's Fay Wray . . .**[1]

## SWOT BOX

- Syphilis was the name of a shepherd infected with the disease in a poem of Fracastorius (1530) perhaps derived from the Greek *syn* (together) and *philein* (to love). It is a subacute to chronic infectious disease caused by a spirochete, *Treponema pallidum*, which appeared in Europe at the siege of Naples (1495). As it spread through the continent, the French called it the Italian disease, the Italians called it the Spanish disease, the Spanish called it the English disease, etc. etc.

- Doctors treated the condition with **quacksalver** (a cream containing mercury). From this we get the origin of the word 'quack'.

- 'You spend one night with Venus and six months with Mercury' was a joke at the time.[2]

[1]Contributed by Dr B. Bhartia.
[2]Source: Liebman, M. Neuroanatomy made easy and understandable, 4th edn. University Park Press; and Dorlands illustrated medical dictionary, 28th edn, 1988, Saunders.

## SWOT BOX *CONTINUED*

- Quacksalver became 'quicksilver', which is still a synonym for the element mercury.

- A **chancre** appears at site of inoculation as a painless **primary** lesion. Described as a small, red papule or crusted erosion, which often breaks down and has a serous exudate (see p. 78 for types of exudate).

- The **tertiary** stage of the illness occurs years after inoculation and can cause many neurological symptoms (neurosyphilis), including **tabes dorsalis** and symptoms such as delusions of grandeur.

- **Tabes** in neurosyphilis is a progressive degeneration of posterior columns, posterior roots and ganglia of spinal cord. Symptoms: lightning pains, ataxia, urinary incontinence, optic atrophy, Charcot's joints, hypotonia and hyperreflexia.

- Transmission may also be *in utero* (the TORCHs mnemonic, see p. 103), leading to various congenital manifestations, including anterior bowing of the mid-portion of the tibia (sabre shin) – a late congenital sign, seen less frequently now due to use of the current treatment, penicillin.

## RUDE RIDDLE

Rude riddle reminder: Why is an Argyll Robertson pupil like a prostitute?

Answer: because it accommodates but doesn't react!

Classically associated with syphilis, it also occurs in conditions such as diabetes and Wernicke's encephalopathy. (Douglas Moray Cooper Lamb Argyll Robertson (1837–1909) was President of the College of Surgeons of Edinburgh in 1886.)

## Tuberculosis treatment

Quadruple therapy is

**RIPE**

**triple therapy:**     **rifampicin**

                        **isoniazid**

                        **pyrazinamide**

**and:**                **ethambutol**

## SWOT BOX

- The usual regimen consists of RIPE for a minimum of 2 months, followed by another 4 months of rifampicin and isoniazid (adults, children and pregnant or breast-feeding women).

- Of course, this also depends on the results of cultures; it may be necessary to increase either or both phases of treatment.

- With CNS involvement the full course is 12 months (RIPE for 2 months + rifampicin and isoniazid for 8 months).

- HIV patients are usually given the standard regime unless multi-drug-resistant TB (MDR-TB) is present. Liver P450 enzyme induction by rifampicin may affect protease inhibitors (makes them ineffective) and an alternative retroviral or anti-TB regimen may have to be used.

- The peripheral neuropathy of isoniazid may be prevented in those at risk (e.g. those with HIV, diabetes, chronic renal failure or malnutrition) by use of vitamin $B_6$, 10 mg daily.

- Poor compliance is best reduced via DOT (directly observed treatment) and the use of combination tablets (e.g. Rifinah®, which is rifampicin + isoniazid), urine testing for rifampicin, etc.[3]

Make notes – it will help you to learn

# Chapter Six

# GENERAL MEDICINE AND PATHOLOGY

*As you read and learn from this chapter you will soon be able to answer all the following, and more.*

## Pre-quiz

- What are the features of acromegaly?
- What are the features associated with carcinoid syndrome?
- Which amino acids are not reabsorbed in cystinuria?
- What are the ECG features of low potassium?
- How would you manage diabetic ketoacidosis?
- Name at least six causes of clubbing.

## Acromegaly[1]

**A**   **arthropathy**

**B**   **big boggy hands**

**C**   **carpal tunnel syndrome**

[1] *Dr Robert Clarke.*

**D** diabetes

**E** enlarged tongue, heart, throat

**F** fields (bitemporal hemianopia)

**G** gynaecomastia, galactorrhoea, greasy skin

**H** hypertension (20–50%)

**I** increasing size of shoes, hat, gloves, dentures, rings

**J** jaw enlarged, prognathism

## Carcinoid

**C** cyanosis

**A** asthma

**R** rubor

**C** cor pulmonale

**I** incompetent tricuspid or pulmonary valve

**N** noisy abdomen

**O** oedema

**I** indoles in stools

**D** diarrhoea

**SWOT BOX**

- Carcinoid tumours are neuro-endocrine in origin and produce a variety of different polypeptide hormones and products especially serotonin (5HT).
- Tumours are generally in the GI tract and are often asymptomatic. Carcinoid syndrome (above) is usually associated with ileal carcinoids because hepatic decarboxylation is avoided.

# Causes of clubbing[2]

| | |
|---|---|
| **Carcinoma** | **e.g. Lung or stomach** |
| **Cardiac** | **Bacterial endocarditis; cyanotic congenital heart disease** |
| **Cervical rib** | **1% of the population have embryological cervical elements which form cervical ribs from C7. A cervical rib may impinge on the subclavian artery and inferior trunk of the brachial plexus and cause neurovascular compression syndrome in the upper limb** |

[2]This version is after A. Ala.

| | |
|---|---|
| **Chest** | **Cystic fibrosis; empyema; bronchiectasis; TB (with extensive fibrosis); fibrosing alveolitis; abscess of lung** |
| **Circulation** | **e.g. A-V fistula in arm (kidney dialysis patients)** |
| **Cirrhosis** | **Check for other signs of liver disease.** |
| **Colonic** | **Crohns; ulcerative colitis; coeliac** |
| **Congenital** | |

Note: 'pseudo clubbing' in thyroid disease.

**SWOT BOX**

Clubbing consists of loss of nail bed angle, increased curvature of the nail (sideways and longways) and increased sponginess of the nail bed.

# More clubbing . . .

## CLUB'D

**C**    **cyanotic heart disease; Crohns**

**L**    **lung disease; liver disease**

**U**    **ulcerative colitis**

**B**    **bacterial endocarditis**

**D**    **diarrhoea (chronic)**

# Cystinuria – COAL

In this hereditary condition, four dibasic amino acids are not reabsorbed by the proximal convoluted tubule (i.e. **cystine, ornithine, arginine and lysine**). The main consequence is that cystine stones are formed in the renal tract (cystine is the least soluble so it forms the stones).

**C**   **cystine**

**O**   **ornithine**

**A**   **arginine**

**L**   **lysine**

Note that cystine stones are seen on X-ray (but are less radiopaque than calcium stones).

# Diabetes mellitus – complications

**KNIVES**

| | | |
|---|---|---|
| **K** | **kidney** | **Diffuse and nodular glomerular sclerosis; uraemia; hypertension; nephrotic syndrome; renal papillary necrosis; atherosclerosis of renal vessels; effects of hypertension** |
| **N** | **neuromuscular** | **Peripheral neuropathy; mononeuritis (see p. 36); autonomic neuropathy; diabetic amyotrophy** |

| | | |
|---|---|---|
| **I** | **infective** | **e.g. urinary tract infection; skin and soft-tissue infection; TB; moniliasis; pyelonephritis** |
| **V** | **vascular** | **Large vessel →; ischaemic heart disease** |
| | | **Small vessel →; microangiopathy** |
| **E** | **eye** | **Cataracts; background proliferative and pre-proliferative retinopathy; micro-aneurysms; maculopathy; fibrosis; retinal detachment; photocoagulation; spots of retinal burns** |
| **S** | **skin** | **Lipoatrophy and insulin sensitivity at injection site; necrobiosis lipoidica; granuloma annulare** |

# Diabetic ketoacidosis – management

I am grateful to Dr R. Clarke of Barnet General Hospital for this suggested scheme pertaining to the emergency management of DKA:

**Think of PANICS to remind you of:**

**P**   **potassium**

**A**   **aspirate stomach (naso-gastric tube)**

**N**   **normal saline**

**I**   **insulin infusion**

**C**   **cultures (mid-stream urine, blood)/catheterize**

**S**   **sub-cut heparin**

# ECG

## ECG and plasma potassium

A lowered plasma potassium level flattens the height of the T-wave.

**Remember: No Pot No Tea!**

## The ECG . . . bundle branch block

With **right** bundle branch block there is an M-shaped wave in V1, and sometimes a W-shaped wave in V6. To remember this, think of:

**V1**    **V6**

**M a R R o W**

and with a **left** branch block you get a W-shaped complex in V1 and occasionally an M-shaped complex in V6:

**V1**    **V6**

**W i L L i a M**

# ECG and heart rates

| 1 | big square = heart rate | 300/min |
|---|---|---|
| 2 | | 150 |
| 3 | | 100 |
| 4 | | 75 |
| 5 | | 60 |
| 6 | | 50 |

# Exudates

**SWOT BOX**

An exudate is material that has escaped from blood vessels or tissues and is characterized by a high protein content. There are six main types: **haemorrhagic, serous, membranous, catarrhal, purulent and fibrinous**.

**'Ham, Sir? Remember Cats Prefer Fish'**

| | |
|---|---|
| **Ham** | **haemorrhagic** |
| **Sir** | **serous** |
| **Remember** | **membranous** |
| **Cats** | **catarrhal** |
| **Prefer** | **purulent** |
| **Fish** | **fibrinous** |

# Favism – G6PD deficiency

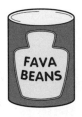

To remember that **favism** [glucose-6-phosphate dehydrogenase (G6PD) deficiency] is associated with **Heinz bodies** in the red blood cell (on blood film, methyl violet stain), imagine a tin of **Heinz 'Fava' Beans**!

## SWOT BOX

G6PD is an enzyme in the hexose monophosphate shunt involved in glutathione reduction. This is essential to protect red blood cell membranes from oxidative crises. If the cell is lacking in reduced glutathione, nothing protects the haemoglobin (Hb) from being oxidized, precipitating rapid anaemia with jaundice.

The oxidized Hb precipitates within the cell to form Heinz bodies, which stick to the membrane making it more rigid. Splenic macrophages lyse the inclusion-bearing cells. This can happen with fava beans (*Vicia faba*), illness, antimalarials or other drugs, e.g. sulphonamides.

# Gait: difficulties in walking

## 'All Patients Spending Cash See Proper Doctors'

will give the important things to consider with abnormal gait. This is explained above (see p. 38).

# Gum hypertrophy

Causes:

**Look, Funny Crowns**

| | |
|---|---|
| **Look** | **leukaemia** |
| **Funny** | **phenytoin** |
| **Crowns** | **Crohns, cyclosporin** |

# Haemophilia

**Haemophilia A** is due to lack of **factor 8**.

**Haemophilia B** is due to lack of **factor 9**.

Think of:

**A ight**

**b = 9 (upside down)**

# HEART SOUNDS AGAIN

## Diastolic murmurs – DAIMS

| | |
|---|---|
| **D** | **diastolic** |
| **A** | **aortic** |
| **I** | **incompetence and** |
| **M** | **mitral** |
| **S** | **stenosis** |

## RAPID REVIEW

Remember 'Mighty Ape' (see p. 54):

| S1 | S2 |
|----|----|
| **M1 T1** | **A2 P2** |

**Mighty Ape**

i.e. **M1 T1, A2 P2**

# Mitral stenosis

According to Rubenstein and Wayne[3] the development of pulmonary hypertension in mitral stenosis is indicated by APRIL:

**A**    **a dominant 'a' wave of the jugular venous pulse (unless in atrial fibrillation)**

**P**    **pulmonary valve second sound is loud**

**R**    **right ventricular hypertrophy**

**I**    **incompetence (i.e. pulmonary – rare), and**

**L**    **a low peripheral arterial pulse volume**

[3]Rubenstein and Wayne 1991: Lecture notes in clinical medicine, 4th edn. Oxford: Blackwell Scientific.

# Heart disease – Secondary prevention

Post myocardial infarct consider:

**ACE ABC**

| | |
|---|---|
| **ACE** | **ACE** inhibitors |
| **A** | **a**spirin |
| **B** | **b**eta blocker |
| **C** | **c**alcium-channel blocker |

# Hepatitis B – the six Hs

**Risk groups** are:

**H**ealth workers (have you had your jabs yet?),

**H**eroin (or other iv drug abusers),

**H**aemophiliacs,

**H**omosexuals,

**H**aemodialysis, and those in

**H**omes (institutions)[4]

# HLA-B27

**Hil-Billies Colliding Sore Ankles are Irate**

| | |
|---|---|
| **Hil-Billies** | **HLA-B27** |
| **Colliding** | **colitis** |

⁴Collier, J.A.B. et al. 1999: Oxford handbook of clinical specialties, 5th edn. Oxford: Oxford University Press.

| **Sore** | **psor**iasis |
|---|---|
| **Ank**les | **ank**ylosing spondylitis |
| are (**R** ) | **R**eiter's |
| **I**rate | **i**ritis (with the Reiter's) |

# Hypertension – causes of

**CREEP**

**C**  coarctation of aorta

**R**  renal

**E**  endocrine

**E**  eclampsia/essential

**P**  pill/phaeocromocytoma

---

## IMMUNOGLOBULIN REVISION BOX:

- We have already seen that the five classes if Ig are 'GAMED' .
- Ig M is produced first in the immune response. Later, Ig G appears as the IgM levels fall. IgG forms the secondary response, which is due to activation of long-lived B cells on repeat exposure to the antigen.
- Ig M is produced IMMediately.

# Lipids again

VLDLs (very-low-density lipoproteins) carry triglycerides from hepatic to peripheral and other cells, where they are stored and later used for metabolism.

HDLs (high-density lipoproteins) carry cholesterol away from the peripheral cells to the liver for excretion.

Think:

**'H for Heroes' and 'V for Villains'**

# Myotonic dystrophy

Popular in exams, this is a rare condition (5/100 000) which often becomes more severe with succeeding generations. Use the first nine letters of the alphabet to help you with some of the main features:

**A**   **atrophy; autosomal dominant**

**B**   **baldness (frontal, in males)**

**C**   **cataracts; chromosome 9 (A–I are first 9 letters of alphabet)**

**D**   **droopy eyes, may be unilateral; diabetes may develop as end organs do not respond to insulin; dysphagia**

**E**   **expressionless . . .**

**F**   **. . . forehead/face (due to wasting of the muscles of facial expression)**

**G**   **gonadal atrophy (small pituitary fossa)**

**H**   **heart (cardiomyopathy and conduction defects)**

**I**   **immunology (low serum Ig); intellectual deterioration**

**SWOT BOX**

- Myotonia is the inability of muscles to relax normally after contraction.

- In advanced disease this is less obvious, owing to muscle wasting. The resulting weakness is the main eventual cause of disability.

- Myotonic dystrophy often manifests in adolescence or childhood and progresses thereafter. There is also an autosomal dominant congenital form (myotonia congenita) which can manifest itself *in utero*.

- During your exam ask the subject to grip your fingers or shake your hand firmly, then let go as fast as they possibly can. The delay in relaxation worsens in the cold and on excitation.

# NEPHROLOGY

## DMSA and DTPA

Two important radiological investigations of renal integrity are the DMSA and DTPA scans:

- [$^{99m}$Tc]DMSA is bound to proximal convoluted tubules in the cortex but gives little indication of the physiological function (e.g. urine production).

- [$^{99m}$Tc]DTPA is given intravenously; a renogram curve shows vascular, secretory and excretory phases.

Highly technical so far, but this helps:

| | |
|---|---|
| **DTPA** | **Does The Physiology** |
| **DMSA** | **Doesn't Move** |

# Cystinuria reminder!

You will already have read earlier that there are four amino acids that are not reabsorbed by the proximal convoluted tubule in this condition: COAL, i.e. cystine, ornithine, arginine and lysine.

# Pain: 'Lost Ward'

Ask about:

**L** location

**O** onset/duration

**S** severity

**T** transmission/radiation

**W** what . . .

**A** aggravates or . . .

**R** relieves

**D** duration/previous diagnoses

## Alternative

**SOCRATES**

**S** site

**O** onset/duration

**C** character

**R** transmission/radiation

**A** aggravates or relieves

**T** timing

**E**   **earlier diagnosis**

**S**   **severity**

# Pancreatitis

## Causes

**GET SMASH'D**

**G**   **gallstones**

**E**   **ethanol**

**T**   **trauma**

**S**   **steroids**

**M**   **mumps**

**A**   **autoimmune disease**

**S**   **scorpion bites**

**H**   **hyperlipidaemia**

**D**   **drugs**

## Investigations

**O, CLAW GUT**

**O**   **oxygen – blood gases**

**C**   **calcium**

**L**   **lactate dehydrogenase**

**A**   **amylase**

**W**   **white cell count**

**G    glucose**

**U    urea**

**T    transaminase**

# Parathyroid glands – all 4s

Here are four interesting facts about these glands:

|                    | **4 glands**                          |
|--------------------|---------------------------------------|
| **Arise from . . .** | **4th (and 3rd) branchial arch**     |
|                    | **40 mg in weight**                   |
|                    | **40 mm in diameter**                 |

## *Secondary hyperparathyroidism – 10 Cs*

**Primary hyperparathyroidism** accounts for 30% of cases of **raised** calcium level:

**bones, stones, moans and abdominal groans**

But in **secondary hyperparathyroidism** the calcium is **lowered**. This is 'coz chronically low plasma calcium levels are the cause of the compensatory increase in PTH secretion. After reading Chapter 8, try coming back to make a 'link' mnemonic for these:

1. Calcium down

2. Cramps

3. Carpo-pedal spasms

4. Chvostek's sign

5. Convulsions

6. Cataracts
7. Cavities (dental)
8. Crazy – change in mental state
9. Cardiac arrhythmias
10. Cranial pressure rises

# Pemphigus

| PemphiguS | Superficial |
|-----------|-------------|
| PemphigoiD | Deep |

---

**SWOT BOX**

- Pemphigus is a group of skin diseases with vesicles and bullae, acantholysis on histology and anti-epidermal autoantibodies.

- Pemphigoid has cleft formation at the dermo-epidermal junction, while immunofluorescence reveals complement and IgG deposits at the level of the lamina lucida of the basement membrane. Yes, you've read it before!

---

# Phaeochromocytoma – '10%'

A usually benign well-encapsulated lobular tumour of chromaffin cells in the adrenal medulla, mainly presents as raised blood pressure (see 'CREEP', in hypertension above). Attacks also cause palpitations, sweating, tremor and nausea.

**10% are multiple**

**10% malignant**

**10% are adrenal bilateral**

**10% extra-adrenal**

**10% are familial**

**10% are in children**[5]

*Alternative: '10% ACME'*

| | |
|---|---|
| **10% are** | **Adrenal (bilateral)** |
| **10% in** | **Children** |
| **10%** | **Malignant** |
| **10%** | **Extra-adrenal** |

# Just in case you skipped the physiology chapter . . . those six anterior pituitary hormones (again!)

'Those Giant Gonads Prolong the Action': the six anterior pituitary hormones are thyroid stimulating hormone (TSH), growth hormone (GH), gonadotrophins (FSH and LH), prolactin and adrenocorticotrophic hormone (ACTH).

| **Those Giant Gonads Prolong the Action** | |
|---|---|
| **Those** | **TSH** |
| **Giant** | **GH** |
| **Gonads** | **gonadotrophins (LH/FSH)** |
| **Prolong** | **prolactin** |
| **the Action** | **ACTH** |

# Rashes and fevers

The following is a guide to which day the rash typically appears after the prodrome, e.g. rubella rash develops on day 1 of onset of fever/illness; scarlet fever on the second day, and so on. Note NO rash is listed at day 6.

**Really Sick People Must Take No Exercise**

| | | | |
|---|---|---|---|
| **Really** | rubella | **Day 1** | |
| **Sick** | scarletina | **Day 2** | |
| **People** | smallpox | **Day 3** | |
| **Must** | measles | **Day 4** | |
| **Take** | typhoid fever | **Day 5** | |
| **No** | | **Day 6** | |
| **Exercise** | enteric fever | **Day 7** | Anon. |

# Raynaud's 'WBC'

WBC gives the colour changes observed in the extremities in Raynaud's, in order:

| | |
|---|---|
| **White** | arteriolar spasm |
| **Blue** | dilated capillaries, skin feels cold, numb |
| **Crimson /red** | reactive hyperaemia as the vasospasm relaxes |

## SWOT BOX

- Raynaud's phenomenon manifests as intermittent ischaemia of the fingers and toes with severe pallor, cyanosis, pain and numbness. It is aggravated by cold or emotional stimuli and relieved by heat, and is secondary to some other abnormality, e.g. systemic lupus erythematosus (SLE), scleroderma, cervical rib, trauma from vibrating tools, beta blockers, ergotamine, oral oestrogens, etc. When the cause is primary, familial or idiopathic, it is called Raynaud's disease. The latter is more common in women.

- M. Raynaud was a French physician (1834–1881); his phenomenon was the subject of his thesis.

# Acute rheumatic fever

## Noodles and Curry on Arthur's Red Cardigan

The five major (Jones) criteria for acute rheumatic fever are carditis (40%), erythema marginatum (10–60%), subcutaneous nodules (10%), arthritis (migratory large-joint polyarthritis – 90%) and Sydenham's chorea (rapid, involuntary, purposeless, jerky movements; L., *chorea*; Greek, *choreia* – to dance).

You might try the mnemonic

## CHANCE

OR, even better, think of Arthur's red cardigan:

| Noodles | nodules |
|---------|---------|
| and Curry | chorea |
| on Arthur's | arthritis |
| Red | erythema |
| Cardigan | carditis |

## SWOT BOX

- The acute systemic illness is due to infection by a β-haemolytic streptococcus, usually between the ages of 5 and 15 years. The heart and joints are mainly affected. The carditis may be myo- endo- or peri-.

- The minor criteria are fever, arthralgia and raised white cell count (FeAR).

- Confirmation of streptococcal infection and two major criteria are diagnostic (or one major and two minor).

- If the attack is severe, or in early childhood or recurrent, the disease may progress to chronic rheumatic heart disease (RHD). It is suggested that there is cross-reactivity between streptococcal and cardiac antigens. Chronic RHD is the largest global cause of heart disease, although less common in developed countries, probably due to the use of antibiotics (the streptococci are susceptible to penicillin).

# Stridor and wheeze

- **Stridor** is a **harsh, grating**, frequently high-pitched breath sound; it is almost always **I**nspiratory, produced by **upper respiratory** obstruction, e.g. in croup.

- **Wheezes** are **polyphonic, high-pitched** sounds, usually caused by **intrapulmonary** airways obstruction. They are usually **E**xpiratory sounds.

So 'I' for inspiratory and 'E' for expiratory. . .

**strIdor**

**whEEzE**

## SWOT BOX: CAUSES OF STRIDOR

- laryngotracheobronchitis (LTB) or croup (parainfluenza type III virus mainly)
- foreign body
- *Haemophilus influenzae* type B infection – epiglottitis (or 'supraglottitis')
- upper respiratory inflammation, e.g. from corrosive, hot, irritant fumes, gases, etc.
- laryngomalacia (congenital floppy larynx)
- congenital vascular ring
- retropharyngeal abscess
- post-intubation
- *Corynebacterium diphtheriae* (diphtheria)
- angio-oedema
- tetany and mediastinal masses

# OPHTHALMOLOGY

## Fundoscopy

Reminder on where to look on fundoscopy:

**DM disc is medial**

**FT fovea is temporal**

## Second cranial nerve: AFRO

A possible scheme if asked to examine the optic nerve would be AFRO:[6]

**A**     **acuity**

**F**     **fields**

**R**     **reflexes (light/accommodation) (NB Do PERLA last, very bright light)**

**O**     **optic disc**

Having examined the optic disc (or 'papilla'), you may see it is choking in fluid ('choked disc' = papilloedema), you will know this from the features CCCP . . .

## Papilloedema – CCCP

**C**     **colour change**

**C**     **contour**

**C**     **cupping, imply . . .**

**P**     **papilloedema**

*With acknowledgements to Dr Lisa Culliford, St Georges' Hospital Medical School.

Make notes – it will help you to learn

# Chapter Seven

# PAEDIATRICS

## Apgar score

A mnemonic used in daily clinical practice all over the world (a great one to show those who tell you they've never used mnemonics!).

**APGAR** stands for **appearance (colour of trunk), pulse, gasp (respiratory effort), activity (muscle tone), and response to stimulation (e.g. irritating the sole).**

|  | Score | | |
|---|---|---|---|
|  | 0 | 1 | 2 |
| **A**ppearance | All over blue | Blue limbs | Pink |
| **P**ulse | 0 | <100 | >100 |
| **G**asp | Absent | Irregular | Regular/crying |
| **A**ctivity | Flaccid | Diminished; limb flexion | Active movement |
| **R**esponse to stimulation | None | Poor, e.g. grimace | Good, e.g. cry |

**SWOT BOX**

- Virginia Apgar (1909–1974) was an American anaesthetist whose name may be the most utilized mnemonic in medicine.
- The score is usually taken at 1 and at 5 minutes after delivery.
- A score of <4 in the first minute indicates that intubation should be considered (especially if the score is falling). Babies with this score have a 17% mortality rate (48% if low birth weight), and if the score is <4 at 5 minutes there is a 44% mortality.

Figures from the *Oxford Handbook of Clinical Specialities*, 3rd edn – which totally overlooks the fact that 'Apgar' is a mnemonic!

# BP in kids

Quick formula is:

$$\frac{90 + \text{age (years)}}{50 + \text{age (years)}}$$

# Breast milk

Advantages:

**B**   **bonding**

**R**   **reduced solutes (compared to formula milk, e.g. less Na, PO$_4$, proteins, etc.)**

**E**   **eczema – lower incidence shown in studies**

**A**   **allergy protection (less likely to develop intolerance to cows' milk protein)**

**S**   **sterilization not required**

**T**   **taurine (aids development)**

**M**   **macrophages kill bacteria**

**I**   **IgA; IQ also higher (due to long-chain fatty acids)**

**L**   **lactoperoxidase; lysosymes and lactoferrrin – promotes lactobacilli, inhibits *E. coli*; long-chain fatty acids (now added to some formulas)**

**K**   **cot death – lower incidence**

*Remember*

**Cows' milk contains Casein – Curd protein**

**Human milk has more wHey**

A milk formula will resemble human milk more closely if it has a higher whey:curd ratio (higher curd formulas are marketed 'for hungrier babies').

# Congenital dislocation of the hip, risk factors – 7 Fs

Congenital dislocation of the hip is associated with:

**First born**

**Female**

**Family history**

**Fetal factors, such as multiple pregnancies**

**Floppy – hypotonia**

**Feet first – more common in breech presentation**

**Freezing – more common in winter-born babies**

# Fallot's tetralogy

**Fella's Blue – Pull his Vest Right Over**

| | |
|---|---|
| **Fella's** | **Fallot's** |
| **Blue** | **cyanotic** |
| **Pull** | **pulmonary stenosis** |
| **VeSD** | **VSD (ventricular septal defect)** |
| **Right** | **right ventricular** |
| **Over** | **overriding aorta** |

**SWOT BOX**

- Fallot's tetralogy was actually first described by Danish anatomist, geologist, Catholic priest and physician to the Italian court, Niels Stensen (1638–1686). He also named the ovary (previously thought of as a female testis), postulating that it was analogous to the egg-laying organ of birds.

- Etienne-Louis Arthur Fallot (1850–1911) was Professor of Hygiene and Legal Medicine at Marseilles.

- Fallot's trilogy is right ventricular hypertrophy, ASD (atrial septal defect) and pulmonary stenosis (RAP).

# Gum hypertrophy: causes

**Look, Funny Crowns**

| Look | leukaemia |
| Funny | phenytoin |
| Crowns | Crohns, cyclosporin |

# Still moping about mumps?[1]

**Meningism**
**Orchitis/Oophoritis**
**Parotitis/Pancreatitis/Paramyxovirus**
**Encephalitis**

[1]These notes are also in Chapter 5 – the more often you read them, the more knowledge you shall have!

**SWOT BOX**

- Mumps is an airborne paramyxovirus (also spread by direct contact via body fluids).

- Uncommon in adults, it is often subclinical in children.

- Usually salivary gland inflammation is the principal manifestation, e.g. parotitis (uni- or bilateral).

- Complications include epididymo-orchitis, oophoritis, meningo-encephalitis and pancreatitis.

- Mumps meningitis is usually benign (vomiting, neck rigidity, lethargy, headache, photophobia, convulsions, abdominal pain and fever).

- Investigations include: CSF, positive throat swab, stool culture and rising titre on serum antibody.

# Nappy rash

**PEE-SAC**

**P**   **psoriasis**

**E**   **eczema**

**E**   **excoriation, e.g. due to diarrhoea, acid stools, disaccharide intolerance, etc.**

**S**   **seborrhoeic dermatitis**

**A**   **ammoniacal dermatitis**

**C**   **candidiasis**

# TORCH'S infections

Important non-bacterial infections that can affect the fetus:

**TORCH**

**T**    **toxoplasmosis (see below)**

**O**    **other sexually transmitted diseases,
e.g. syphilis (see p. 66)**

**R**    **rubella (an RNA virus)**

**C**    **cytomegalovirus – see below**

**H**    **herpes, e.g. chickenpox**

**S**    **slapped cheek (parvovirus B19)**

## *Cytomegalovirus (CMV) – 3s*

**3**

**3%**    **is the rate of primary infection
(making this the most common
primary infection in pregnancy)**

**30%**    **risk of transmission to fetus (half of
these are due to reactivation of the
virus)**

**3**    **per 1000 births, UK incidence[2]**

[2]*Figures from Gilbertson and Walker* Notes for the DCH, *1st edn. Edinburgh: Churchill Livingstone.*

## SWOT BOX: CMV

- 95% of affected infants are asymptomatic – although 10% of these may become deaf in later life. There is a 30% mortality rate for those with severe congenital disease.
- Complications include low birth weight, neurological sequelae, abortion, anaemia, hydrops, pneumonitis, purpura.
- Investigations: CMV on throat swab/urine/infant serum IgM.
- Transfusion services provide CMV-screened blood for neonates.

## *Toxoplasmosis –'tOXO' tetrad*

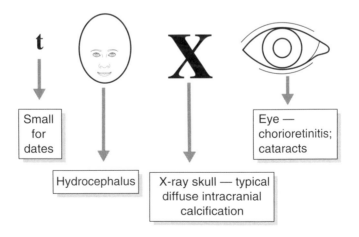

t → Small for dates

Hydrocephalus

X-ray skull — typical diffuse intracranial calcification

Eye — chorioretinitis; cataracts

## SWOT BOX: TOXOPLASMOSIS

- The protozoan *Toxoplasma gondii* has its sexual cycle in the cat; it enters the human food chain by ingestion of oocytes, e.g. via raw meat from other animals.

- 75% of the UK population are susceptible to this; however, the vertical transmission rate is only 1:1000 and only 10% of affected fetuses are damaged.

- Infected patients may be totally asymptomatic or may develop a non-specific illness with fatigue and flu-like symptoms.

- 12 cases are reported annually to the CDSU (Communicable Diseases Surveillance Unit).

- Pregnant women found to have seroconverted may be treated with three-weekly courses of spiramycin to reduce risk to the fetus. Infected neonates may be treated with spiramycin alternating with pyrimethamine + sulfadiazine.

Make notes – it will help you to learn

# Chapter Eight

# SURGERY AND STUFF

*A sprinkle of urology tips and a few sieves to boot . . .*

## Pre-quiz

- Describe the branches of the renal artery.
- What should you ask in the history of a person with jaundice?
- What are the X-ray features of Crohns?
- Who traditionally are said to get gallstones?
- What are the risk factors for congenital dislocation fo the hip?
- What are the signs of an arterial thrombus?
- What features on a mole imply a high suspicion of malignancy?

## Surgical sieves

Two olde favourites:

**In A Surgeon's Gown Physicians Might Make Some Progress**

| | |
|---|---|
| **In** | incidence |
| **A** | age |

| | |
|---|---|
| **Surgeon's** | **s**ex |
| **G**own | **g**eography |
| **P**hysicians | **p**redisposing factors |
| **M**ight | **m**acroscopic |
| **M**ake | **m**icroscopic |
| **S**ome | **s**urgery |
| **P**rogress | **p**rognosis |

**In A Surgeon's Gown, A Physician Can Cause Inevitable Damage To Patients**

| | |
|---|---|
| **In** | **i**ncidence |
| **A** | **a**ge |
| **Surgeon's** | **s**ex |
| **G**own | **g**eography |
| **A** | **a**etiology |
| **P**hysician | **p**athology |
| **C**an | **c**linical; presentation |
| **C**ause | **c**omplications |
| **I**nevitable | **i**nvestigations |
| **D**amage | **d**ifferential diagnosis |
| **T**o | **t**reatment |
| **P**atients | **p**rognosis |

## *'VITAMIN C DIP' sieve for aetiologies of pathologies*[1]

Completely daft but it works something like this:

**V**    **vascular**

**I**    **infective**

**T**    **trauma**

**A**    **allergy/immunological**

**M**    **metabolic/endocrine**

**I**    **iatrogenic**

**N**    **neoplastic**

**C**    **congenital**

**D**    **degenerative**

**I**    **idiopathic**

**P**    **psychogenic**

# Abdominal distension – 6 Fs

## A Flatulent Fat Fetus floats in Fluid Faeces

[1] By Dr Bobby Bhartia, St Georges' Hospital Medical School.

# Arterial thrombus: 'P' signs

**Pale/pallor**

**Painful**

**Pulseless**

**Paralysed**

**Paraesthesia**

**and Perishing with cold!**

# Burns – the rule of 9s[2]

| | |
|---|---|
| **BACK OF TRUNK** | **9% × 2** |
| **FRONT OF TRUNK** | **9% × 2** |
| **EACH ARM** | **9%** |
| **EACH LEG** | **9%** |
| **HEAD and NECK** | **9%** |
| **Perineum** | **1%** |
| **Hand** | **1%** |

NB Do not include simple erythema in the estimate.

# Congenital dislocation of the hip, risk factors – 7 Fs

Congenital dislocation of the hip (CDH) is associated with:

[2]Collier, J.A.B. et al. 1999: Oxford Handbook of Clinical Specialities, 5th edn. Oxford: Oxford University Press.

**First born**

**Female**

**Family history**

**Fetal factors, such as multiple pregnancies**

**Floppy – hypotonia**

**Feet first – more common in breech presentation**

**Freezing – more common in babies born in winter**

## CROHNS – the X-ray

You need to know the following characteristics features of a Crohns on X-ray:

**C**  **cobblestone appearance of mucosa**

**R**  **rose-thorn ulcers**

**O**  **obstruction of bowel**

**H**  **hyperplasia of mesenteric lymph nodes**

**N**  **narrowing of lumen**

**S**  **skip lesions/(sarcoid foci/steatorrhoea)**

# Gallstones – 5 Fs

**Fair**

**Fat**

**Female**

**Forty**

**Fertile**

# Haemorrhoids: clover leaf

Analogous to a clover leaf at positions 3, 7 and 11 o'clock . . .

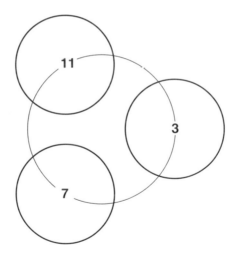

External haemorrhoids are varicosities of the inferior rectal vein tributaries.

# Jaundice – the history

When taking a history from somebody with jaundice you may find the mnemonic CATHODES helpful:

**C**    contacts

**A**    anaemia

**T**    travel

**H**    had it before

**O**    operations

**D**    drugs (including iv recreational use)

**E**    extrahepatic causes (e.g. gallstones, sickle cell )

**S**    sexual preference

# Kyphosis and scoliosis

Kyphosis anterior curvature of the spine

Scoliosis lateral curvature of the spine

# Management: TIE

If ever stuck in an OSCE or viva on a question of how to manage a case, a useful tip is TIE:

**E**  **explanation to the patient**

**I**  **investigation**

**T**  **treatment**

*While there is tea, there is hope.*
*Sir Arthur Pinero (1855–1934)*

# Meckel's diverticulum – rule of 2s

This is part of the vitello-intestinal duct which completely disappears in 98% of the population. It causes complications such as perforation, haemorrhage from peptic ulceration, obstruction (as it contains cells similar to those from stomach or pancreas). A Meckel's diverticulum occurs:

**in 2% of the population**

**2:1 is the male:female ratio**

**2 inches long,**

**2 feet from the iliocaecal valve on the antimesenteric border of the small intestine**

## SWOT BOX

J.F. Meckel the Younger (1781–1833) studied medicine at Vienna and discovered the first branchial cartilage. His grandfather first described the spheno-palatine ganglion and his father was a Professor of Anatomy and Surgery.

# Melanoma

## ABCD; BITCHES

**(1)**

| | | |
|---|---|---|
| **A** | **ASYMMETRY** | irregular |
| **B** | **BORDER** | notched, indistinct or ulcerated |
| **C** | **COLOUR** | increasingly variegated, especially black/grey |
| **D** | **DEPTH** | of invasion |

**(2)**

**B** **BLEEDING**

**I** **ITCHING (persistent)**

**T** **TETHERING**

**C** **COLOUR**

**H** **HALO**

**E** **ECZEMA-LIKE FEATURES**

**S** **SIZE (rapidly increasing)/SATELLITES (presence of)**

# Prostatic hypertrophy

A quarter to half of all men in their 40s and 50s have benign prostate hypertrophy[3]

[3]Data from Forte and Vincent. Ten tips of treating enlarged prostate. Doctor Magazine, June, 2000

**(think of 1/4 to 50% of men aged 40–50)**

**60% of men in their sixties**

**70% of men in their seventies**

**80% of men in their eighties**

Get it?

# Sprain treatment – RICE

A very commonly used mnemonic in clinical practice by many health professionals.

**R**  **rest**

**I**  **ice (or cold pack, e.g. frozen peas, gel packs, etc. If using ice, crush it, wrap it up in layers of towelling; apply for 10–15 minutes, not directly on the skin. If using peas, do not eat them, mark the bag with a big 'X' to avoid possible food poisoning!)**

**C**  **compression (tubular crepe bandage)**

**E**  **elevation (keep the affected limb elevated)**

# See also

1.  Renal arteries, p. 7.

2.  Cystinuria, p. 75.

3.  DMSA, DTPA, p. 85

Make notes – it will help you to learn

# Chapter Nine

# OBSTETRICS

## First, FORCEPS . . .

**F**    fully dilated

**O**    occiput presentation

**R**    ruptured membranes

**C**    catheter to empty bladder

**E**    engaged

**P**    pain relief should be adequate

**S**    space/scissors (episiotomy)

## Which forceps – WAK

| Cavity | | Forceps |
|---|---|---|
| low | **W** | **Wrigley's** |
| mid | **A** | **Anderson's** |
| high | **K** | **Kielland's (rotational)** |

Of course, the use of ventouse has largely superseded the high-cavity forceps.

# Causes of ante-partum haemorrhage (APH)

**A**  **abruption**

**P**  **placenta praevia (or vasa praevia)**

**H**  **hardly known – 40% are idiopathic**

# Pelvic dimensions – 11, 12, 13

The 11, 12, 13 'rule' helps to give you the approximate ideal female pelvic dimensions. These are approximate anterior–posterior dimensions.

The variation in diameter through the pelvis is a human characteristic – an adaptation to bipedal stance – it helps one walk upright but makes the second stage of labour more difficult for the fetus, which has to rotate the head to negotiate the varying shape of the pelvic 'tunnel'.

**11 cm (antero-posteriorly) × 13 cm (transversely)   PELVIC INLET, going in is wider transversely**

**12 cm, mid cavity of pelvis   MID CAVITY**

**13 cm (antero-posteriorly) × 11 cm (transversely)   OUTLET, coming out is wider antero-posteriorly**

# Sperm counts – guide to the norms[1]

Think of the sequence **2, 2, 4 ,6** because a normal sperm count may be considered to have the following normal values:

[1]Anon. but apologies to Norm . . .

| Minimum count | **20 million,** |
| in | **2 mL** of which |
| at least | **40% are motile, and** |
| at least | **60% have normal morphology** |

# Sterilization counselling

**FEMALE**

**F** failure rate (1 in 500)[2]

**E** ectopics (small relative increase in risk)

**M** menstrual changes (such as not taking the pill any more)

**A** ain't reversible

**L** laparoscopic procedure (may be done at Caesarean section if baby is healthy)

**E** enter in notes ('informed of failure rate, knows irreversible')

[2]Collier, J.A.B. et al. 1999: Oxford Handbook of Clinical Specialities, 5th edn. Oxford: Oxford University Press.

# TORCH'S infections – a reminder

Important non-bacterial infections that can affect the fetus:

**T**  **toxoplasmosis (see p. 104)**

**O**  **other sexually transmitted diseases, e.g. syphilis (see p. 66)**

**R**  **rubella (an RNA virus)**

**C**  **cytomegalovirus – see below**

**H**  **herpes, e.g. chickenpox**

**S**  **slapped cheek (parvovirus B19)**

## *Cytomegalovirus (CMV) – 3s*

**3**

**3%**  **is the rate of primary infection (making this the most common primary infection in pregnancy)**

**30%**  **risk of transmission to fetus (half of these are due to reactivation of the virus)**

**3**  **per 1000 births, UK incidence[3]**

[3]Figures from Gilbertson and Walker Notes for the DCH, 1st edn. Edinburgh: Churchill Livingstone.

## SWOT BOX: CMV

- 95% of affected infants are asymptomatic – although 10% of these may become deaf in later life. There is a 30% mortality rate for those with severe congenital disease.

- Complications include low birth weight, neurological sequelae, abortion, anaemia, hydrops, pneumonitis, purpura.

- Investigations: CMV on throat swab/urine/infant serum IgM.

- Transfusion services provide CMV-screened blood for neonates.

See also Syphilis, p. 66.

Make notes – it will help you to learn

# Chapter Ten

# ADVANCED MNEMONICS

*Introducing the 'memory training' concepts of association; conquer those cranial nerves; use the power of pegs; and a session on the link.*

## ASSOCIATION

> *In the first place, Association*
> > Harry Lorayne and Jerry Lucas 1996:
> > The memory book. *Ballantine Books.*

This is the process that links the new fact/word you *want* to learn with information that you *already know*, e.g. numbers, the alphabet, members of your family, your bedroom, etc.

We know that the nature of brain pathways are such that any word or thought can link you to a myriad of other words (see your neurology texts). In fact your brain works in a non-linear fashion, like a mind-map.

Take for instance the word 'chocolate' – immediately many mental associations can come to mind. If you channel your thoughts in this direction, almost instantaneously you will generate literally hundreds of thoughts, ideas, words, connotations, mental images, memories and so on. And you do all of it in milliseconds while being totally relaxed and laid back about the whole experience!

So if your brain already works this way naturally, why not make use of this to *deliberately* associate new facts to things you already know?

You can repeat a fact to yourself until your brain gets the message and creates a link by the random way (like how long will that take!) – *or you can make it easier.*

There is nothing new about association, it was a used by the ancient Greeks to memorize key words in their long orations. They would take a mental tour around their homes having already associated key concepts to objects they already knew. After all, you remember where your bed is and what your bathroom looks like. The phrase, 'In the first place', is said to come from this. This is the loci memory system. This technique is still used now by speech-makers and memory experts and is great for learning Krebs cycle in a hurry.[1]

Making associations deliberately is done by using *mental pictures.* You need to exercise your imagination by producing vivid, exaggerated mental pictures, evoking strong imaginary emotions and made as ridiculous and out of place as possible. If you have made it this far, you already have the skills to learn a few 'advanced' memory tricks!

For instance if a pigeon flew overhead yesterday lunchtime, chances are you won't even have remembered it. But if an elephant with a striped hockey stick and yellow polka dot boxer shorts flew over your head, you would most likely remember that image for the rest of your life. You may also remember what day it was and what you were doing at the time.

Make your imaginary pictures extreme, exaggerated, ridiculous, bold, funny and outrageous (it's OK – it's all in your head!).

---

### GOLDEN RULE

Ask yourself, *'If it happened in real life, is it something I would always remember?'* (e.g. Martians land in your back yard). You see, you can make it up *and it will be just as memorable.*

---

# THE POWER OF THE PEG – AND THOSE CRANIAL NERVES

Having delved into the world of making associations with extreme pictures, we can try simple 'peg'. Peg methodology involves a minimal

[1] *In fact, there will be more on this, with examples, in the next edition of this book.*

effort initially, but enables you to learn lists easily and reliably in and out of sequence.

To do this you have to know how to count up to, say, 12. (Peg systems exist that can go up into the thousands.)

First, spend the next *60 seconds* memorizing the following list:

**1.** run

**2.** shoe

**3.** tree

**4.** door

**5.** hive

**6.** sticks

**7.** heaven

**8.** gate

**9.** dine (or 'line')

**10.** hen

**11.** level crossing (or 'leaven')

**12.** elves (or Twelfth Night)

Done it?

Here we have learnt a system for using *images* to code for *numbers*, making visualization easy.

We begin associating our list to the 12 pairs of cranial nerves. You don't have to use my suggestions – your own pictures will work even better.

# Cranial nerve I is olfactory

Imagine say, an oil factory (oil refinery or perhaps an oil drilling platform). These are *substitute* words to help you remember the word 'olfactory'. Using substitutes facilitates visualization of vague terms.

So the 'oil factory' will be your analogy for the first nerve. Meanwhile, you know that a substitute word for ONE is RUN.

Now add movement – see, for instance, this oil factory growing enormous legs, like an ostrich or a dinosaur, and RUN down your street as fast as its huge, gangling, creaking bulk will allow. Close your eyes for a moment to let that picture crystallize clearly in your mind. Involve all of your senses, smell that crude oil (it is the first nerve after all). See splodges of oil being shaken off and landing all over the place. Feel the ground shudder with each step.

We have now associated **one** with **olfactory**. Easy enough? So let us travel to TWO, which in our system transposes to SHOE.

# Cranial nerve II is optic

Two codes to shoe. One can visualize wearing SHOES instead of glasses (optics). Or maybe smashing a pair of optics by stamping on them with your favourite, newest, most expensive shoes. See the vivid image, now exaggerate it beyond belief – make those optics shatter into millions of pieces which fly up and gather into a whirlpool of whizzing optics while you shoe continues on relentlessly . . .

# The third nerve is the oculomotor

Imagine a TREE with motorized branches; at the end of each branch is an eye (oculus). The eyes are clicking and whirring on those motorized branches, all focusing and staring at you – hundreds of motorized eyes looking straight into yours, and yet you have an unusual feeling of well being as you realize these are your creation, entirely safely within your mind's oculus, with you in total control. Make the motorized branches dance and whirl as they click and spin. Got the picture? If not make up another!

# IV is the trochlear nerve

We use DOOR to represent the numeral four. Not just any door, but one meaningful to you, e.g. your own front door or that of somebody close to you.

Substitute words for trochlear may be truck, trog, etc. (or even a pulley if you know that *trochilia* is Greek for a pulley). The possibilities are now limitless! Well, you might see a truck with a pulley ripping off your front door while you watch in horror and disbelief, or you might see yourself being hauled up the door by a large pulley, etc. etc. Whatever you decide, make the image bright, bold and noisy, and exaggerated in every sense.

# Nerve number V is the trigeminal

The substitute word for five is HIVE. You may, for instance, visualize an enormous hive, but instead of bees or wasps imagine of lots of precious gems buzzing around the hive; see them whizzing in and out and flying about your ears as the gems sparkle and shine. You might even imagine three such hives or make the hives look like three giant gemstones. Make it so ridiculous and out of place that *had you seen it in real life you would remember it forever.*

Alternatively you can use the word 'Gemini' (for trigeminal) and imagine say, triplets instead of twins, and then link the triplets to a beehive.

Use whatever forms your association in the easiest most memorable way.

# The sixth cranial nerve is abducens

SIX transposes to STICKS. You can use a simple picture, such as abducting your arms with a big stick, although in this case make the picture vivid. Feel the stick jagging against your arms as they force them outwards. Feel the texture of that hard unforgiving stick! OK, OK, so make up your own, why don't you!

# The seventh cranial nerve

The number SEVEN is HEAVEN and the seventh cranial nerve is the facial nerve.

You can visualize graphically many faces, including your own, falling down from the sky (heaven). See in detail the expressions on these millions of faces as they keep falling down relentlessly. Large faces, small faces . . . also perhaps imagine cloud-shaped faces floating in the sky, perhaps laughing, some of them frowning, some smiling, etc.

# The eighth cranial nerve

We now need to link the number eight (GATE) to the vestibulocochlear nerve. So, see a gate in your mind, not just any gate but a gate of importance to yourself, such as your own front gate, or perhaps on a building you admire. On that gate you can perhaps hang/impale all your favourite vests (or perhaps you can see lots of gates wearing vests, dancing in and around as in a 'Gap' clothes advert).

Alternatively, you can see a giant ear in place of the gate, and you're pushing this ear away in order to get through the gate.

# The ninth cranial nerve

Let's link number nine (DINE) to the glossopharyngeal nerve. Although you should have the hang of it by now, one suggestion would be to have a giant pharynx being dined upon – at a very glossy dinner party. Give the giant pharynx a good dose of pharyngitis – hear its hoarse sound, make it look so very sore and phlegmy.

# The tenth cranial nerve

Number ten is HEN. See an enormous hen perhaps laying an egg – make the hen look suitably vague for 'vagus' (or dressed like a magus). Maybe a hen on the cover of *Vogue* magazine or a hen in Las Vegas. Or whatever you fancy.

# Eleventh cranial nerve

Number 11 can be called LEAVEN. It is difficult for some people to visualize (leaven is yeast that makes bread rise). You can also visualize a LEVEL CROSSING to represent the number 11.

This is the accessory nerve. You decide on the type of accessories you will use here. Then envisage all of your favourite accessories being crushed under several high-speed trains. See trains hurtling past on the level crossing as to you try to dash in and out between them in order to retrieve your precious accessories . . .

# The twelfth cranial nerve

Twelve rhymes with ELVES. Then imagine a dozen elves with giant tongues hanging out. Perhaps they are all experiencing hypos, because they are unable to eat due to the size of their giant tongues. This should be sufficient to remind you of the hypoglossal nerve.

*IMPORTANT: Now run through those silly images two or three more times in the next couple of minutes.*

So now we have:

| | |
|---|---|
| **run** | **olfactory (see the mental picture you made)** |
| **shoe** | **optic** |
| **tree** | **oculomotor** |
| **door** | **trochlear** |
| **hive** | **trigeminal** |
| **sticks** | **abducens** |
| **heaven** | **facial** |
| **gate** | **vestibulocochlear** |
| **dine (or line)** | **glossopharyngeal** |
| **hen** | **vagus** |
| **level crossing (or leaven)** | **accessory** |
| **elves** | **hypoglossal** |

Run this list through your head a couple of times, then backwards. We are ready for a test!

- Which is the seventh nerve?

Think of number seven; see the picture that you imagined (e.g. faces in the sky).

Note how you link this picture to what represents a . . . *facial* nerve. And you **know** it is the *seventh* nerve. *How cool is that?*

OK, try these . . .

- Which is the seventh nerve?
- Which is the eleventh nerve?
- Which cranial nerve is the oculomotor?
- Which cranial nerve is in the abducens?
- Which is the first cranial nerve?
- Which number is given to the trigeminal?
- Which is the third nerve?
- Which is the twelfth nerve?
- Which is the facial nerve?

Looks like you have got the hang of it! Incidentally even if you didn't stop and review things along the way as instructed (and I'm pretty sure you didn't), you would still have got most of these correct.

Congratulations, you now know the cranial nerves in and out of order, and you know the number assigned to them, also in and out of order.

You did this with ease and loads of fun. Just review a few more times now in order to cement them into your long-term memory.

PS After using this several times you will no longer require the actual mnemonics.

You can use the same substitute word numbers for any other list you like. However, I will suggest another list to use for something else, this time involving visualization of similar objects rather than rhyming words.

1. A pencil (looks like the number 1)

2. Swan (looks like number 2)

3. Stool (with three legs)

4. Table with four legs (or a square window)

5. A five-pointed star

6. A yo-yo hanging from string

7. The seven dwarves

8. An octopus

9. Lollipop

10. A spoon placed to the left side of a round plate

11. Twin Towers/chimneys

12. A dozen eggs

13. Baker's dozen; Friday the 13th, etc.

As an exercise, why don't you spend the next 5 minutes using the new easy way to memorize some key facts relevant to bronchial carcinoma:

1. men (more common in)

2. malaise and anorexia

3. haemoptysis, shortness of breath, recurrent infections

4. Horner's syndrome (related to site of invasion)

5. Pancoast (likewise)

6. intracranial metastases

7. neuropathy and proximal myopathy

8. malignant hypocalcaemia

9. dementia

10. cerebellar ataxia

11. polymyositis

12. HPOA (hypertrophic pulmonary osteoarthropathy including clubbing, periostitis)

13. acanthosis nigricans

You can, of course, associate anything to anything, so you can use the parts of your own body, your friends, etc., on which to 'peg' facts.

# THE LINK: MAKE ASSOCIATIONS WORK FOR YOU

'Linking' is a good way to learn sequential lists. For instance, let us suppose you want to learn a list of words, like:

- Triad

- Muffins

- Heart

- Big jug

- Hypo

Imagine a group of three Hong Kong gangsters (triad). Now make a ridiculous picture of them all swathed in enormous muffins that are so exaggerated they are being choked and muffled by these huge muffins. Make that image vivid and colourful; give it sound, feel the crumbs, smell the freshly baked essence of those muffins as they swallow up our triad gangsters whole. We need an exaggerated picture, so make sure there are thousands of these giant muffins. Give them flavour, e.g. chocolate.

This links triad to muffins.

Now from muffins, think of 'heart'. Perhaps you can see muffins pumping blood around your body, or a heart squeezing out fragments of muffins in systole, with each beat the crumbs being forced out and getting shredded . . .

Now from 'heart' go to 'big jug'. Link the two word-pictures in an incredulously silly fashion, e.g. pouring hearts out of a giant jug into your drink; watch them slide out of the big jug and land with a sickening 'glunk' in your glass. They are actively pumping oxygenated blood and there seems to be an endless supply.

Or perhaps you can think of another way to link pumping hearts to big jugs.

Finally link jug to 'hypo'. Let us say, for instance, that your jug is now empty and you have to fill it using a whopper of a hypodermic syringe; gasp as the jug gradually fills and develops a smile on its face . . .

How do you remember that this is the *final* item on the list? Simply link it either back to the first item, making a loop, or perhaps to a fixed reference image, e.g. your own feet.

Now just think of 'triad' (again you can use a fixed reference image, such as your own head, for the start). This will make you think of the picture related to 'muffins'. Muffins remind you of 'heart'. Heart links to 'jug' and finally this associates with 'hypo'.

This sounds a bit iffy I know, but at least you have learnt *Beck's triad of pericardial tamponade*, as well as how to use a linked list. (The triad is muffled heart sound, raised jugular venous pulse and hypotension. OK, you did not really need all the above to do this, but the intention is to illustrate the technique.)

*NOW . . . Try making a link for something else, e.g. the 10 Cs for hyperparathyroidism in Chapter 6.*

Using your own pictures will be more effective. (Fortunately, most medical students are good at daydreaming.)

# THE LOCI SYSTEM

Essentially this uses the positions of things to learn lists, facts, biochemical cycles, etc. As mentioned earlier, the loci system was used by the ancients and is my favourite method of learning lists. It is intended that there will be more on this powerful system in the next edition . . . see you there!

*Imagination is more important than knowledge.*

*Albert Einstein*

Make notes – it will help you to learn

# Chapter Eleven

# REVISE AT THE MOVIES!

## MORE LINKS AND LOCI

In the Chapter 10 you learned that memory consists of linking what we want to know with what we already know – and as you can associate anything to anything else, it is possible to use your favourite movies, soaps and sporting events, etc. to revise. People often remember their favourite movie or sporting event in remarkable detail – why not put this to good use?

We will explore how to make use of a memory we already have to learn something we need for our exams!

NOTE: Unlike the rest of this book, this chapter may be more difficult to follow if you have not read the previous one.

I have decided to use as our example *The Wizard of Oz* (by L. Frank Baum), purely on the assumption that it is likely to be familiar to all or most readers. (Hey, stop complaining – or in the next edition it will be the *Sound of Music!*)

If you somehow have managed *not* to see this film, then go and watch it now – it is essential for your revision!

OK, you already know how to link memories consciously, i.e. associate them to something you already know by means of exaggerated use of your imagination. (If not, go and read the last chapter you skiver! Honestly!)

Make use of movies/events/football teams, etc. that you are already know by heart. The more detail you know, the more facts you can associate into your key scenes/characters/players/sportsmen, etc.

So what to learn?

As an example, just for the heck of it, why not learn the *peripheral somatosensory system pain and temperature pathway*? As these pathways are quite awkward to learn, you may as well get them out of the way now.

*You can use any other list or topic you wish* (remember this book is your willing slave and not the other way round!). Here goes . . .

# PERIPHERAL SOMATOSENSORY SYSTEM PAIN AND TEMPERATURE PATHWAY

- **Receptors** are in the dermis/ epidermis of skin (arranged in overlapping **dermatomes**).

- Sensory neurons travel to **dorsal root ganglion** (a few branches will travel up or down a segment and enter the dorsal horn at a different level – this allows *overlap*).

- The nerve synapses in the **dorsal horn** of the spinal cord.

- The second (post-ganglionic) neuron now **crosses** over to the contralateral side in the **ventral white matter**;

- then it **ascends in the lateral white matter**.

- Remember that from the synapse in the dorsal horn mentioned above there are also some short secondary internuncial neurons that connect with motor neurons to form the **reflex arc**.

- Back to the collection of crossed fibres going upwards (via the internal capsule), they are known as the **lateral spinothalamic tract**,

- they travel to the **thalamus**, where they

- synapse in the ventral posterolateral nucleus (**VPL**).

- Tertiary neurons now go to the **postcentral gyrus** (area 3,1,2) of the cortex. This is the main somatic sensory area of the brain.

I have selected a few key words here – once we have a group of key words you can begin constructing a mnemonic-based memory aid.

Back to *The Wizard of Oz*! We need the key events from the story. Briefly,

- Dorothy lives on a farm in Kansas with her dog, Toto
- House is blown away up into a tornado
- House crash lands in Oz
- Munchkins
- Enter Glinda the Good Witch
- She gives Dorothy a pair of ruby slippers
- Dorothy follows the yellow brick road where she meets
- The scarecrow who wants a brain
- Tin woodman who needed oiling and wants a heart
- Cowardly lion
- They have a nice snoozy time in a field of scarlet poppies (quite advanced I thought for a kiddies movie, but then maybe I am showing my age!)
- Emerald City – they have to wear emerald glasses
- They meet the Wizard who sends them off to defeat the Wicked Witch of the West
- They travel through the dark enchanted forest
- They are carried to the horrible witch by winged monkeys
- Dorothy melts the witch with a bucket of water
- Oz turns out to be a fake wizard with a big balloon
- Dorothy clicks her heels together to get home

OK, now all you need to do is link what you need to know with what you already know (*Wizard of Oz*). *I have put in one or two suggestions but now you have to do a little dream-work* (more fun than normal work). Once you have learned the principle, you can use this with other movies, soaps, the FA Cup final, World Cup 1966, etc.

| What you know already | Facts you need to learn | Dream-work; suggestions – but make your own notes |
|---|---|---|
| Kansas, farm | Pain and temperatures | E.g. very hot on farm (exaggerate the picture beyond belief!) |
| Tornado | Start with pain and temperature in the dermis | Tornado blows off all of Toto's and Dorothy's dermis and epidermis |
| Crash land | Dorsal root ganglion | Crash on back of (dorsum) of a gang of Munchkins? Make the pictures vivid, put in sound, colour and sensations . . . |
| Munchkins | | ditto |
| Glinda, ruby slippers | Branches overlapping up/down a level | So many slippers that slippers overlapping with her shoes |
| Yellow brick road | Synapse, dorsal horn | If you haven't read the previous chapter by this stage you may be a little lost – go back now! |
| Scarecrow | Crossing over | Make your own images, make them outrageous and whacky |
| Tin man | | |
| Lion | | The rule is one movie per mnemonic! |
| Scarlet poppy field | Ascending in the lateral white matter | etc.! |
| Emerald City | Short neurons form the reflex arc | |
| Wizard of Oz | Lateral spinothalamic tract | |

| What you know already | Facts you need to learn | Dream-work; suggestions – but make your own notes |
| --- | --- | --- |
| Dark forest | Thalamus | |
| Winged monkeys | Synapse in VPL | |
| Witch melting | Postcentral gyrus | |
| Bogus wizard flies off in balloon | Near the central fissure | |
| Click heels three times | Area 3,1,2 | Dorothy counts 3,1,2 as she clicks her heels. She is a bit divvy and gets the numbers out of order . . . |

# HOMEWORK!

OK, now you are getting the hang of it:

1.  Write a list of possible mnemonic lists, e.g. movies you know well.

2.  OR . . . watch as many movies/sporting finals, etc. that you love, or videos of sporting events (DVDs if possible, as pausing the scene is easier).

3.  Now a list of events you know really well, e.g. weddings, football matches, hockey finals, etc.

4.  You can do this with routes too, e.g. the route on your way to college – you may have done it hundreds of times and know it backwards! (This is the loci system again – more in the next edition.)

5.  You can do this with lists you already know, e.g. your flatmates, characters in your Bridge Club or whatever.

6.  Pick a few topics in which sequences are important and dig out those *key words* – this is one of the most important stages because it makes you *summarize and review* as you do so. And you will remember that summarizing and reviewing are the two most important revision skills, regardless of how you do them.

7. Make a table as above, jot down in rough pencil your mental imagery. Or you can use a mind map.

8. When revision time comes you will only need to revise the mnemonic and not pile through pages of text, a serious time-saver for 'night-before' revision!

9. Enjoy!

Make notes – it will help you to learn

# Chapter Twelve

# MOTIVATIONAL BITS, QUIPS AND STUDY TIPS

*A pot-pourri of thoughts, ideas and wisdom, ancient and modern, together with a soupçon of solidly useful study tips to see you on your way . . .*

Suddenly the euphoria of being at university is gone; there is an eerie silence in the air; where once there was laughter and milling throngs, all around is despair. And worst of all, the weird sensation that even though surrounded by hundreds of other people, you are almost alone . . . yep, it's exam season again!

Well, like I said, almost alone – now is the time you find out who your friends really are – and you will have discovered that this little book is up there with the best of them!

So put the kettle on, strap yourself into that chair/couch/bed, and be prepared to share some wisdom from some of the world's finest thinkers – and as you meld in this way, remember that you, too, are amongst them!

*The surest way to be late is have plenty of time.*

*Leo Kennedy*

# How common is common?

Try this if stuck for figures:

| | |
|---|---|
| **1:30** | **common** |
| **1:300** | **uncommon** |
| **1:3000** | **rare** |

# Breaks

Have regular breaks! So how do you have a break?
  Say, for a full day's study:

- Start off with a 10–20 minute break each hour when you are fresh.

- Be flexible with your breaks – with experience your own body will tell you what feels right.

- Then as the hours pass by and your interest starts flagging, you may need to increase the break times in order to keep studying efficiently.

- So by the evening you may have half an hour swotting followed by half an hour's break.

- Before you start your break, run through what you have just done in your mind for a few seconds only – so you skim through main headings and points at high speed.

- When you come back from your break, rapidly skim through, in your mind's eye, the stuff you did previously, for another few seconds – this sets you up quickly to get back into 'mode'.

This way, in any 12-hour period you will get several hours' productive revision done. Working flat out without a break only gives you useful revision for the first few hours, after that you become tired, may lose interest and your learning starts to flag. Twelve hours straight without a break is very inefficient compared with the same period with realistic, generous and regular breaks.
  Don't forget to eat as well as having tea/coffee breaks.

# Caffeine

Certainly extremely useful as a mild stimulant – beware of overdoing this though, as it can only give you so much of a lift before the shakes start, diuresis (not helpful during exams) and, even worse, diarrhoea and wind (not helpful to the person in the chair behind you).

Too much sleep deprivation is also unhelpful, and remember that caffeine may stay in your system for hours, so even when you do sleep it will reduce the overall quality of your sleep and may give you that 'why am I tired all the time if I am having loads of caffeine?' syndrome. Be good to yourself. And set realistic goals.

# Goal setting

- Define your study goals/amounts/times before you start.

- Give yourself *realistic targets* – learn smarter. Time is limited (both for you and your swotty neighbour). If it won't help you pass, then ignore! Emerson said 'Life is too short . . .!'

- Also define your *break times* (see above, p. 144), a 'countdown timer' is useful – found on most digital watches, microwaves, PDAs and kitchen timers, etc.

    *Allow for 2 minutes' overview at the beginning of your sessions and 5 minutes reviewing at the end of your sessions.*

- So decide what you will learn *now* and what you will cover later (when, and if, you have the time). This is called prioritizing your resources and it is an especially important skill for doctors.

- Define goals for the session; the day; the term; a year or even your lifelong targets. The use of goals, targets, etc. has permeated all walks of life, from fiscal to political, motivational, self-development, etc., for the simple reason that goal setting works. Write down your goals/aims/objectives, etc.

    *'If you have some definite goals in mind your thoughts will help to take you there and you will tend to be dwelling on your goals. If you have no goals your*

*thoughts will facilitate you towards what you think about most.'*[1]

- However, if your dominant thoughts are of a football match, movie, going out, etc. – good news!! *It is still possible to mnemonic these events by associating them to the facts you wish to learn* (see Chapter 11).

- Fill your thoughts with images and visions of yourself making the *exam* suffer for using up so much of your time . . . aim for an elegantly detached matter-of-fact state, where there is just enough adrenaline and sympathetic activity to keep you alert and interested.

## SMART goals are:[2]

**S**   **specific and simple**

**M**   **measurable and meaningful**

**A**   **all relevant areas**

**R**   **realistic and responsible**

**T**   **timed toward what you want**

- According to Edison, genius is 1% inspiration and 99% perspiration.

- Many of your colleagues are saying that they have not done any work. Well, what they mean is that they have not done as much as they like (and have actually done more than they realize – or are prepared to admit).

- This is a common phenomenon in the medical schools game because the selection process seems to pick out many pathological perfectionists . . . they could never have done enough work and rely on denial as a bizarre motivational strategy.

[1] *Andrew Matthews 1988:* Being happy! A handbook to greater confidence and security. *Media Masters.*
[2] *In various sources, this version adapted from Tad James 1988:* Time line therapy and the basics of personality. *Wood Meta Publications.*

- This is fine because different people work in different ways. Your task is to recognize this and accept it. Nobody knows as much as you think they do – and you know more than you realize!

- Remember – nobody knows everything. Walter Mondale said 'If you think you understand everything that is going on, you are hopelessly confused.' Make your learning efficient and ecological. Pay particular attention to your learning environment.

# Environment

Learning is a process by which you brain makes certain neurological connections. Everything happening to you at the time you learn adds a few sub-branches to that particular connection in your neural network (see any neurology text).

So if you are doped up on caffeine while revising, your brain remembers that too. When you need to reproduce the information in your exam with no caffeine in your bloodstream, the brain will find it that much harder to access the facts you need. Thus psychologists describe learning as being 'state specific'. (You may have heard about students who could only pass exams while having raised blood ethanol levels and who are useless while sober – now you know why.)

In other words, match every aspect of your environment – including biochemical – to simulate as near exam conditions as possible. If possible, you can even revise the subject in the room you are taking the exam in.

If not, then you can use different rooms for different subjects (then thinking of the room, remembering what it looks and feels like will act as memory joggers). This also helps reduce confusion between subjects.

Emulate your blood levels of caffeine and glucose to simulate what you will experience during the exam. If music helps you remember, and if you are not allowed to wear personal stereos during the exam, then beware! (If no other option, listen to it on the morning of the exam). Take whatever sensible and logical steps you can – then go for it!

# Go for it

*whatever you can do, or dream you can . . . begin it.*
*Boldness has genius of power and magic . . .*

*Goethe*

*'Make It So!'*
   *Captain Jean-Luc Picard from* Star Trek, the Next Generation

*People wish to learn to swim – at the same time to keep one*
*foot on the ground.*

*Marcel Proust*

# Good . . .

*To the good, be good:*
*to the bad be good too – in order to make them good as well.*
                 *TheHe Zhizhang, Tang dynasty*

*The good is the beautiful.*

*Lysis*

*If you cannot speak good of someone, be silent.*
                 *Reported by Bukhari.*

# Key facts

You are aware of the concept of 'key words/facts' or phrases – to put it simply, those facts that will give you *marks* in the exam.

   Once you have gained an understanding of a topic, don't spend time learning anything unless it can be classed as directly relevant to obtaining exam marks. Once exams/assessments are no longer an issue of course, you can learn as many irrelevant facts as you wish! And have a good laugh about it. Even better, laugh all the way through your revision too.

# Laughter

*'When the first baby laughed for the first time, the laugh broke*
*into a thousand pieces and they all went skipping about, and*
*that was the beginning of fairies.'*

*Peter Pan*

# Map and territory

*The map is not the territory.*

*Korzybski*

# Mind maps

*Use mind maps*. Invented by Tony Buzan decades ago, they are surprisingly underused. Many of you will have come across them from school.

Mind maps are especially useful for previewing a topic at the start of the study session, reviewing at the end, and for making essay/project plans.

They are very useful for an exam with lots of sections or written parts – you start off several mind maps, one for each section. Then start writing your answers. As you write, the earlier questions serve as memory joggers and ideas will come for the later parts. You can immediately jot these down on to your other mind maps.

If attempting to answer a question you know nothing about, doodling with a mind map can glean some answers from the inner recesses of your unconscious mind!

Your space for a mind map:

# Morning before

OK, so you have got up, ideally having had a few hours sleep to let yesterday's revision sink into longish-term memory. Have breakfast! (Unless you have done all of your learning on an empty stomach – see 'Environment', above.)

If you used caffeine during revision, then have one cup of whatever you used, now. Skim through your cards/summarized notes and mind maps and *mnemonics*. Reinforce material you have covered previously.

It makes sense to have at least an hour of mental relaxation just before the exam, to let everything sink in and assimilate, allowing your neurotransmitter levels to recharge. You will need them at their peak to blitz these exams.

# Night before

It is usually better to get a few hours of quality sleep the night before – the rare exception is when you only have a single exam to do and really have done no preparation whatsoever. Having worked efficiently with plenty of breaks (see 'Breaks' and 'Environment'), you should be tired enough to get to sleep. The day/night before is usually when your mnemonics are most helpful (that is why we have kept this book portable).

However, if you have a string of exams, etc. to sit, over a period of several days, simply staying up all night will turn you into a zomboid amnesiac as you stare blankly at your exam paper.

While you sleep your mind keeps working, sorting and assimilating what you have learned. If you stay awake all night learning lots of last-minute minutiae, you will certainly remember what you have just read in the last 2 hours or so (short-term memory) but are equally likely to have forgotten much of the earlier stuff. You decide if the trade off is worth it (very occasionally it is).

# Problems?

*Nothing lasts forever – not even your troubles!*

*Arnold Glasgow*

*. . . the problem is not the problem; the problem is the way people cope. This is what destroys people, not the problem.*

*Then when we learn to cope differently, we deal with the
problems differently – and they become different.*

Virginia Satir

*. . . the package deal in being human involves problems and it
means we get to love, to laugh, to cry, to try to get up and fall
down and to get up again.*

Andrew Matthews

*The way I see it, if you want the rainbow, you got to put up
with the rain.*

Anon

*The mud puddles of life are only there to remind you it's just
been raining.*

Stan Lee

*Obstacles are things a person sees when he takes his eyes off
his goal.*

E. Joseph Cossman

*It is no good crying over spilt milk because all the forces of the
Universe were bent on spilling it.*

William Somerset Maugham

*If opportunity doesn't knock, build a door.*

Milton Berle

# Patients and preparation

*To study medicine without reading textbooks is like going to
sea without charts, but to study without dealing with patients
is not to go to sea at all.*

Sir William Osler (1849–1919, said to be the most outstanding
medical educator of his time. Said to be a man of immense
personal charm, he is also credited with introducing bedside
teaching to medicine.)

*The secret of patient care is caring for patients.*

Peabody

# Principle of precession

According to the principle of precession, by Buckminster Fuller, we gain many things on the way, in addition to the actual goal itself.

The important thing may not be reaching the goal, but how much we learn as we go along the way.

The journey is as important in many ways as the piece of paper you are getting at the end.

*The mirror reflects all objects without being sullied.*

*The heart of the wise, like a mirror, should reflect all objects without being sullied by any.*

*Confucius*

Confucius probably did not intend a mirror to be a revision aid, but you can write on it with washable ink or stick on a Post-it® note – *one* fact per mirror– which you never think about again, but as you look at the mirror each day it will become etched indelibly into your long-term memory (passive learning).

# Record cards and Post-it® notes

Post-it® notes are quite a handy way of learning complex topics, by breaking them down into smaller parts. The advantage of using them is that they can be arranged in different ways over books, notes, walls, bathroom mirrors, doors, wallpaper, etc.

Don't have more than one or two facts per Post-it® note – *keep it simple* – avoid visual indigestion. Likewise, only have two or three Post-it®s per mirror/door, etc. (or posters even). (A whole wall with dozens of Post-it®s is an inefficient, time-consuming, re-hashing process, although it may impress your flat-mate!) Within reason, of course, you can do whatever you like.

You can use the same Post-it® notes later as *bookmarks* in different textbooks – which allow you passively to review the diagram, fact, etc., even while you simultaneously study a completely different topic (neat, huh!).

Record cards can be used in a similar way.

As time is limited, once you've put the topic/facts on record cards (or Post-it® notes) you should avoid duplication (yawn) by making yet more notes on those same facts. Instead, maximize remembering those facts on your cards, etc., by any means necessary.

You can use your revision cards while walking, waiting for the bus, in the dentist's waiting room, etc. Their convenience lies in their portability. Remember that one or two clear, bold facts/diagrams/mind maps per card is enough.

# Review, review, review

The single most important study secret. You will notice that reviewing is the fundamental ingredient of all revision strategies.

So how does one review? Any way you like; although a few useful ways are to spend a few minutes (no more!):

- either scribbling down a mind map (2 min);

- or visually scanning over the material in your mind's eye;

- or flicking through your Post-it® notes or record cards.

- You can even go through your textbook/notes again – provided you only look at (quickly) the facts you have highlighted or underlined, etc.

So when should you review? Ideally:

- At the start of your session do a quick, mental, 2-min overview of what you know of the topic – even if you think you don't know anything. It is permissible to look at past papers/previous years' tasks instead.

- After every paragraph or every few key facts (if paragraphs are irrelevant).

- At the end of the session do a quick 2-minute visual fast forward in your mind, like scanning on a video.

- After 24 hours.

- After 1 week.

- After 1 month.

- Pre-exam (this is usually the only time anybody else does it!).

Reviewing like this takes effort and seems to slow you down – but all this reviewing doesn't mean you need to spend hours slogging through lots of facts. Once you have gone through the material initially, you only need to review your key words, facts and phrases.

# Regular breaks

We know that it is more efficient to study in sessions of 20–40 minutes and to take regular breaks (e.g. 10–20 minutes). Yep, we have talked about breaks earlier!

As well as keeping up your energy levels by taking breaks, the chance to share ideas and mnemonics with your friends, breaks allow you to *review* the stuff you have just learnt and to *overview* the stuff you are going to learn. Do this at the beginning and end of your study sessions.

Many find they get their best ideas and brainwaves when most relaxed, e.g. in the shower, loo, bed, etc. When you relax you go into an alpha-wave state, where you are at your most creative.

> *We have the best results in our life when we are prepared to go with the flow. This means finding the delicate and elusive balance between effort and relaxation, between attachment and letting go . . . Relax and let go – go with the flow.*
>
> *Andrew Matthews*

# Reward

> *The highest reward for a person's toil is not what they get for it, but what they became by it.*
>
> *John Ruskin*

# Smile similes

> *Smile, it'll increase your face value;*
>
> *Smile and the whole world will smile with you;*
>
> *Smile – it'll squeeze out endorphins from those reluctant neurones;*
>
> *'Coz you smile when you feel good,*
> *And you feel good,*
> *When you smile.*
>
> *Various*

# Staggering sessions

This does not refer to what you do on your way back from the medical school bar!

Staggering sessions means that you *alternate your subjects*. Study at least two topics at one sitting and make sure these are as dissimilar as possible. So, for instance, study anatomy for an hour or so, then alternate with sociology and then biochemistry and then back to anatomy.

You'll keep your mental energy levels up this way, while covering the same volume of material – and retain more. This is because you'll avoid the fatigue associated with boredom. This gives those crucial neurons in the relevant section of the brain an hour's rest before returning back to the original topic – as we know that different memories, different subjects, use different sections of the brain. It is thus useful to know a variety of study methods.

# Study methods

Use any combination of study methods and keep them flexible!

Studying (like medicine) is really more of an art than a science. There are no absolutes! Be as flexible as you like . . . *so long as you take regular breaks and review frequently,* really any study method will work.

Suggestions include Tony Buzan's Organic Study Method. This has defined stages, including overview, preview, in-view, review, etc. This way you cover the topic several times, looking at different aspects and different levels of detail each time. Other versions include SQ3R (survey, question, read, recite, revise), etc.

The secret is to find the most appropriate method for you, for that topic, for that time and for that place – *as long as you take regular breaks and review often*.

# Sticky wicket?

*Man who removes a mountain begins by carrying away small stones.*

*Chinese proverb*

*Common sense is genius dressed in its working clothes.*

*Emerson*

*Success is more attitude than aptitude.*

*Anonymous*

*Failure lies not in falling down but in not getting up*

*Traditional Chinese proverb*

*Life can only be understood backwards;*
*but it must be lived forwards.*

*Søren Kierkegaard*

*Experience, the name men give to their mistakes.*

*Oscar Wilde*

# Small is beautiful!

- *Small is beautiful* in the world of MBBS revision – get the smallest book on the topic. You always have lots of other information sources available, e.g. tutorials, handouts, friends, internet, etc.

- Only use the *minimal number of books* per topic – a standard text, a crammer and a revision Q&A type book is probably still too much (but I will forgive you!).

- *Study groups* can delegate workload to different students – you then teach each other – a terrific way to cover large amounts of material in a short time.

# Summarize

It has been said that you know you have learnt a topic if you can condense a huge wodge of notes down to the size of a postage stamp!

In practice, if you can summarize all the material from one subject into a few pages/cards, etc., you can be sure you will have understood the material. Then you only need to memorize the key facts. These key facts can be put on to a mind map for at-a-glance overviewing/reviewing.

Effective summarizing explains the popularity of finals revision courses which condense the whole MBBS clinical course into a weekend – with good results.

So summarize, summarize your summary, then summarize that. Then teach it to your colleagues and let them return the favour on another topic you don't have time for.

# Taking yourself too seriously

It is only an exam!

Keep things in perspective. Are you filling your mind with gloomy thoughts? What a waste! This is a symptom of taking yourself too seriously!

If you want to exaggerate and magnify vivid thoughts in your mind, make sure they are of nice things in the world around you, all the positive things that have happened and will happen. Or of fabulous mnemonics to learn things quickly and laid back! And if you are really convinced you will re-sit, then continue to revise anyway as you will still need to learn the stuff and any exam practice will be useful (you may even pass . . .).

If you are really desperate to be serious about anything, 'be serious about humour!'

*But it does move.*

*Galileo*

# Texts are tools

Your texts are your tools and your servants – not the other way around!

It is better to get your own books and highlight, <u>underline</u>, make notes in the margin, cross out waffly paragraphs, whittle the words down to what is useful *now* to *you*.

Doing all this will help you learn.

A lot of the excess words are there to help you understand; many wasted words in those big books are the writer's personal view of the universe – forget all that! Remember what you need to help you gain useful knowledge in the most useful way to get marks . . .

The text is *your* slave!

*We get taught a lot of things that are never useful.*

*Richard Bandler*

# Winnie the Pooh

*While Eyeore frets and Piglet hesitates and Owl pontificates . . .*

*Pooh just IS.*

*Benjamin Hoff in* The Tao of Pooh

# Wisdom and knowledge

*One of the greatest pieces of economic wisdom is to know what you do not know.*

*John Kenneth Galbraith*

*Can your learned head take leaven*

*From the wisdom of your heart?*

*Lao Tse (translated by Witter Bynner)*

*And finally . . .*

*They know enough*

*who know how to learn.*

*Henry Adams*

Enjoy!

Make notes – it will help you to learn

# INDEX

162